AS YOU WERE

VE Day: a medical retrospect

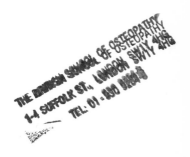
Published by the British Medical Association
Tavistock Square, London WC1H 9JR

The extract from *Who's Who* on the back cover is reproduced by permission of
A & C Black Ltd.

British Library Cataloguing in Publication Data

As you were: VE Day: a medical retrospect
1. World War, 1939–1945—Personal narratives
940.54′81   D811.A2

ISBN 0–7279–0181–8

Filmset and printed in Great Britain by
Latimer Trend & Company Ltd, Plymouth

Preface

It was Max White who in February 1984 suggested that the *BMJ* should commission a series of memories by doctors of their experiences on D Day, wherever they were at the time, and publish a book on its fortieth anniversary in June dedicated to the memory of Elston Grey-Turner. Not even the *BMJ*'s contributors, and its printers, can work as fast as that, however, but another idea came up: to link the memories to VE Day, almost a year later, and invite our contributors to range widely about their wartime experiences. This we have done and the result to me is a marvellous and revealing book. It is still dedicated to Elston's memory, and, given the tributes paid to him here, especially Sir Ferguson Anderson's address at the memorial service, I will add little more save to say that he was a splendid colleague, tolerant and supportive, and to thank all those who have contributed their accounts.

STEPHEN LOCK
Editor
British Medical Journal
November 1984

Contents

Glossary

ADMS Assistant director of medical services

AOCME Air officer commanding middle east

Asdic Device for detecting submarines (from Allied Submarine Detection Committee)

ATS Auxiliary Territorial Service

CCS Casualty clearing station

C in C Commander in chief

CMF Central Mediterranean Force

CO Commanding officer

CRA Commander, Royal Artillery

DADMS Deputy assistant director of medical services

DDMS Deputy director of medical services

DGMS Director general of medical services

DMS Director of medical services

EMS Emergency Medical Service

FSU Field surgical unit

FTU Field transfusion unit

GHQ General headquarters

GOC General officer commanding

HQ Headquarters

HQME Headquarters middle east

In the bag Taken prisoner

LIAP Leave in addition to python

MO Medical officer

NAAFI Navy, Army and Air Force Institutes

NCO Non-commissioned officer

NMA Netherlands Military Administration

OC Officer commanding

OTC Officers' Training Corps

PMO Principal medical officer

POW Prisoner of war

Python End of a period of overseas service, and leave then granted

QA Queen Alexandra's Imperial Military Nursing Service

RAMC Royal Army Medical Corps

RASC Royal Army Service Corps

RCAF Royal Canadian Air Force

RMO Resident medical officer

RNVR Royal Naval Volunteer Reserve

RSO Resident surgical officer

SEAC South East Asia Command

SHAEF Supreme Headquarters Allied Expeditionary Force

STC Senior Training Corps

TA Territorial Army

TD Territorial (Officer's) Decoration

VAD Voluntary Aid Detachment

Future assured

ROBERT M ADAM

When VE Day came I was a midshipman on a battleship of the British Pacific Fleet, and our thoughts were firmly set on the grim battles that we were sure would come in the final invasion of the home islands of Japan. It was therefore in many ways rather a non-event in the fleet. We had been told that there were going to be extra rations of canned beer and of course the main brace was spliced for the sailors, but for some reason our beer never got through to us and I remember it as being a very routine day.

It had been my life's ambition to join the navy. Originally I had hoped to go to Dartmouth, but my parents were against this and so as soon as I was old enough I left school and joined the navy under the Y scheme, which allowed me to go to Cambridge as an undergraduate on a short course, combining it with naval training. After Cambridge I went to sea as an ordinary seaman, then, with the rest of my contemporaries of the university naval division, to HMS *King Alfred* in Hove, where we were commissioned – most of us as midshipmen as we were under 19½. On leaving the *King Alfred* some two dozen of us were despatched immediately to the Pacific to join the growing fleet preparing for the final battles of the war.

As a boy I read voraciously all the books I could get my hands on about the navy, and was brought up on a diet of "Bartimeus" and "Taffrail". I do not think anyone was keener than me to serve as an officer in the Royal Navy. My father, who is a general practitioner, gave me some very sound advice before I finally left school. From his experience in the first world war, when he had seen large numbers of men returning to universities and the fierce competition for places, he advised me to put my name down for a medical school before I went to sea, and I am eternally grateful to him for

1

his advice. How different it was in those days getting into medical school from the problems the students tell me they have to face today. When the Dean at Barts, the late Sir Gerling Ball, heard that I was asking for a postwar place my interview lasted for approximately another 15 seconds: he said, "Father a doctor – delighted my boy!" shook my hand, and I was out of his office. So I went off to sea with the comforting thought that if I survived my future career was assured.

Preparing revenge

In 1941 and 1942 we had been humiliated by the Imperial Japanese Navy. The *Prince of Wales* and *Repulse* had been sunk off Malaya, and in the battle of the Java Sea the famous *Exeter*, the victor of the River Plate, had also been sunk. The proud Royal Navy had been swept out of far eastern waters and at one time the remnants of our fleet even had to retreat as far west as Mombasa for a base. Our hold on Ceylon was precarious, and the Japanese very nearly succeeded in invading it in 1942. Nevertheless, the Royal Navy had hung on and was determined to be in the last battles against the Japanese to revenge our humiliation.

Against what we now know to have been considerable opposition from the Americans the British Pacific Fleet was built up, using Australia as the main base. What a marvellous experience it was to be there as a 19 year old after six years of wartime England with its blackout and rationing restrictions. The lights, the fruit, the girls, the unbombed streets, the bronzed and healthy people living normal lives virtually untouched by war, apart from their men serving overseas – what a time we had. There was enormous unbounded Australian hospitality: parties, picnics, beaches; attempting to learn to surf; trips into the Bush. To my sorrow for various reasons I have not yet been able to return to Australia but my memories are as vivid as ever after 40 years.

Preparations were being made for the main battle ahead. Okinawa was conquered by the Americans with our fleet acting as support. Our carriers were in action and everyone was aware of the fanatical courage shown by the Japanese and their incomparable airmen, so patriotic that they were prepared to kill themselves as kamikaze pilots in the defence of their sacred homeland. We knew that in the final battles we would have to face them and many more. We were also aware of the Japanese home army of some three million or more men who had not yet fired a shot in anger, who were prepared to fight to the last man in defence of their emperor. We all viewed the invasion to come with a considerable degree of apprehension.

The news of the falling of the first and then second atom bomb came to us as a marvellous relief. The development of the atom bomb was, of course, the war's best kept secret, although interestingly enough I had wondered why a young scientist I knew at Cambridge suddenly disappeared to go to America on secret work at very short notice. I knew he was a physicist and we guessed that they were developing something very special, so special it would be dangerous to produce it in England.

Saved by the bomb

The news of Japan's surrender made us wild with joy. I have seen pictures of the scenes in London on VE Day, but I am sure they cannot have been any more wild or enthusiastic than those which took place in Sydney on that day in August 1945. Not only had we won the war – we had survived. Our prisoners would be coming home and not massacred as we had expected had we invaded Japan. Life would return to normal; we would take up our chosen careers; and we really did think there would never be another war.

I continued to serve for nearly another two years before demobilisation and had most interesting experiences serving in the far east. We left Australia, went to Singapore, and soon after the surrender of Singapore saw our prisoners come out of Changi. I had six months on loan to what was then called the Royal Indian Navy and saw something of that magnificent country. I remember the great professional satisfaction of learning my job as a naval officer, learning to take command, to keep watch at sea – and one of my proudest possessions is still the full watch keeping certificate I earned.

Eventually, of course, we came home. It was really a "Cook's tour", stopping at every naval port between Singapore and Rosyth. I hung up my uniform with many regrets and put on my sports jacket to be a medical student and become immersed in the grind required for the first MB. I still feel that I am one of those who survived the war almost certainly because of the atom bomb, and I could never be a unilateral disarmer. God forbid there should ever be another world war, and I pray that the world will be spared the

3

horrors of nuclear annihilation. Nevertheless, I remain convinced that without the bomb the war would have dragged on for many more months, there would have been hundreds of thousands of Allied casualties and unknown numbers of Japanese. President Truman's decision to drop the bomb has been strongly criticised in many circles but not, I know, by any of us who served in the British Pacific Fleet 40 years ago.

Travels on the all red route

MELVILLE ARNOTT

I recall a recruiting poster of long ago which had as its caption the phrase, "Join the army and see the world". My army service fulfilled amply this promise. From mobilisation on 1 September 1939 to 30 September 1945, when I left Redford Barracks with an ill fitting "demob" suit, I had ranged from the Great Wall of China to the Harz Mountains in Upper Saxony. Some 20 different countries intervened.

How did it all start for me? As a fairly senior territorial officer, first in the Royal Artillery and then the Royal Army Medical Corps, I was posted to the command of a training company at the depot. A few weeks later I was told that the War Office had phoned to say that Arnott or another officer at the depot was to go to China as a medical specialist, leaving in 72 hours – embarkation leave had not yet been invented. Such incidents illustrated well the jolly, haphazard way in which Britain went to war. My friend and I sat down over a drink to decide which of us was to go. We were both very attracted by the prospect and eventually we settled the matter by the toss of a coin. Arnott was for China. I had just time to have a tropical uniform run up, purchase a copy of Rogers and Megaw's *Tropical Medicine*, and bid farewell to my bride of a few months, whom I was not to see again for four years.

The wrath to come

It was a tedious journey, first across France to Marseilles and from there by "slow boat to China" in the ancient troopship *Nevassa* – coal burning, with a maximum speed of 12 knots. The Union Jack still flew the world over and it was an all red route – Malta, Egypt, Aden, India, Ceylon, Malaya, and Hong Kong. Leaning over the

5

rail, looking at a scene of tropical splendour, somebody remarked that in peacetime people used to pay big money to see this sort of thing. "Yes," came the retort, "but they had a return ticket – we haven't." Sad memories of shipmates who never needed a return ticket.

I was sent as medical specialist to the British Military Hospital in Shanghai, combined with duty as medical officer to the Seaforths. The international settlement was guarded by British, American, and Italian troops. All around the Sino-Japanese war was raging and refugees were crowding in to the settlement. Corpses in the street were a common sight. But the lifestyle of the Europeans remained undisturbed, unbelievably prosperous and hedonistic. With the fall of France it seemed painfully obvious that Japan would follow Italy by declaring war on the West. British outposts in Peking, Tietsin, Shanghai, and Hong Kong would be quickly overwhelmed. Two of us planned, when the crash came, to escape up the Yangtze River. Once in Chinese Nationalist territory, as doctors, we hoped to earn our rice. In August, however, came the code signal "Pacific", which meant evacuate north China. I was sent to accompany the Peking and Tietsin garrisons to Shanghai and travelled by coal boat to Chin-Wan-Tao, where the Great Wall of China comes down to the sea, and then onwards by train – probably the last British officer to travel in uniform on the Mukden–Peking express.

I saw the Union Jack lowered in Tietsin and later in Shanghai – "Sic transit gloria". I went with the Seaforths to Malaya while others went to Hong Kong, where in due course they died or were captured. It was an anxious journey south. We were shadowed by Japanese warships, there was a nearby typhoon, and the Japs had mined all the typhoon anchorages.

Malaya seemed singularly unperturbed, with little apprehension of the wrath to come. The *Aedes* mosquito was ubiquitous and dengue was epidemic. I caught it and found it a very unpleasant illness, aptly named by Benjamin Rush "breakbone fever".

Audacious exercise

After some months I was posted to the middle east and on the way visited the Institute of Tropical Medicine in Kuala Lumpur. There, Dr Field, the distinguished malariologist, gave me the formula of his rapid thick film stain. This I handed over to Brigadier Neil Hamilton Fairley in Cairo. It was quickly put to use.

There followed busy months in Jerusalem, surely the world's most memorable city. I had the wonderful experience of treading the Via Dolorosa on Good Friday. The Syrian campaign brought many more medical casualties than wounds: malaria, enteric, dysentery, relapsing fever, and diphtheria. I received a small supply of the new drug sulphaguanidine, which I gave, with miraculous results, to a Free French officer dying of Shigella dysentery.

One day there came an order to move, and I was on the advance guard. It was the prelude to an audacious exercise. We moved with great secrecy to Alexandria, joined a mixed force, and made a highspeed dash on destroyers and a cruiser, reaching Tobruk on a moonless night having dodged air attacks. We scrambled up the cliffs, achieving for me the greatest physical exertion of the war. There is nothing like a bit of shot and shell to unlock reserves of energy. We got in comparatively unscathed but subsequent assaults were disastrous, with loss of a cruiser, destroyers, and many men.

Our hospital was in only moderately damaged buildings. There were frequent air attacks and continuous desultory shelling. As sieges go it was not too bad. There were considerable stocks left by the Italians, and although we were chronically hungry and lost much weight we were not starving. Ample supplies of ascorbic acid tablets prevented scurvy. Water was very short and brackish as the wells were being overpumped. I must confess that several months without a bath in unwashed clothes proved remarkably tolerable. When the siege was lifted and I went aboard a hospital ship I was shepherded downwind and ushered to a bathroom.

Desert sand is remarkably free of pathogens, permitting "primary suture" with little sepsis. Among memories is that my boots wore out completely, but when I was literally down to my uppers I noticed, projecting from under a blanket, a pair of boots on the feet of a casualty who had died as he reached us. The "dead man's shoes" were a perfect fit. Another time, playing bridge, I opened with a heart; this was followed by a spade. There then intervened the scream of an approaching shell. There was a crash, darkness, and then from the far corner of the room my partner, in a squeaky voice, called two clubs.

Retreats and disasters

Most of 1942 was disastrous. With the retreat to the delta and Stalingrad I doubted if I would ever see my native land again. For a short time I was attached to a medical research unit to study wound shock, but we found it very difficult to catch up with the cases as desert warfare is so mobile. We spent much time digging our trucks out of the sand. Much of 1943 was spent in Palestine with 23 (Scottish) General Hospital and a medical division of 1200 beds occupied mainly by cases of infective hepatitis.

During this time I had an unpleasant reminder that I was aging in the service of my king. I was rejected as too old at 33 for parachute training with a view to dropping into Yugoslavia to help the partisans. I had to be content with playing a small part in training a group of young chaps for the job.

In November I was posted to the UK and travelled by Sunderland flying boat, masquerading as a civilian, via Tunisia, Gibraltar, Lisbon, and Shannon, coming down in Poole harbour. These were great moments – setting foot on Britain and being met in the middle of the night by my wife at Princes Street station, Edinburgh.

I am afraid I was a latecomer to the invasion. Ostend had just been captured when I landed and joined a hospital at Duffel. On VE Day itself I happened to be at GHQ in Brussels when the definite news came in of the signing of the Act of Surrender. I hurried back to Duffel with the glad tidings and the town was soon en fête. We arranged a grand reception attended by the local notables. Enough good cheer was found to make everybody happy. Within a few days I was on my way through the shattered Ruhr to a hospital near Hannover. I saw Belsen and it brought home to me the horror of the evil force we had subdued.

My experience of warfare was more directly concerned with retreats and disasters than victories but the one predominant memory that stays with me is the indomitable courage of the British soldier. The British people are at their best in adversity and at their worst when "never having had it so good".

*   *   *

I did not come to know Elston Grey-Turner until after the war, but held him in the highest esteem and affection. It would have been a privilege to have served with him.

Cakes and ale

C E ASTLEY

I joined the RAF about a year after qualifying at Leeds, on the advice of a friend who recommended it as a piece of cake and not much to do; said he: "It would suit you a treat, Cliff." So, being single, I sent in my application. Looking back I now see that he held this view in a very quiet period of the war, called at the time the phoney war – it just hadn't really got going in western Europe. My second house job ended conveniently a few weeks before I was called up to report to RAF Halton, near Aylesbury, where medical entrants gathered for two weeks' instruction in RAF matters and methods, plus some square bashing and being instructed how to salute, something I had previously learned at OTC. I arrived at Halton on 11 June 1940; shortly afterwards France fell and I recall the gloom and depression this cast upon us all. I also remember the time taken in instructing us on a piece of Heath Robinson like apparatus called the water cart. This contraption had a huge tank for water and lots of gauges and dials and glass tubing. I think that if properly used it would produce clean from unsafe water over-seas, but so complicated did it appear that few of us really understood it. I thought it would be bad luck if I ever saw one again – my bad luck arrived some two years later.

Pleasant trip

After Halton I was posted around the UK for 18 months on ground training stations; it was an unremarkable period, though it did much to improve my snooker. Then in December 1941 someone must have decided to get rid of me and I was posted to the middle east. After a sad goodbye to my parents and fiancée, who flatly refused to marry me then, I sailed down the Clyde in the

Viceroy of India on 12 January 1942 and started writing my diary. We were a big convoy with lots of troop ships and merchant vessels, the battleship *Resolution* and some six destroyers flanking the convoy far out. I remember walking round the decks endlessly as we sailed out west, always counting the ships, and one day a troop ship was missing; we heard it had been struck by a torpedo, but it managed to limp into the Azores, then Gibraltar.

Apart from this incident the journey was uneventful and as we moved into warmer weather so did we begin to enjoy ourselves. The *Viceroy* was very comfortable, with much of its peacetime trimmings including, in the officers' mess, a lovely grand piano which we used for concerts; there seems never to be a dearth of entertainers among troops, most of whom on this ship were army, but we also had quite a number of RAF doctors posted to Cairo to open a new RAF hospital there. I could never see the need for this, but shrank from saying so, not wishing to be friendless the rest of the trip. I remember we ate and drank heartily, played bridge for hours most days and worked up to duplicate. We read the supplied literature on tropical medicine, and twice daily we had the radio news on the BBC overseas (now world) service. By the time we reached Freetown we were nicely tanned. It was hereabouts the blackout was lifted; we were not allowed ashore, but I shall never forget hearing the choir from the *Resolution* singing "Over the sea to Skye", so well did the sound travel over the quiet harbour water. After Freetown the convoy stopped the zigzag course so we moved faster; at the Equator we did not omit the ceremony of crossing the line, and I was thrown into the pool with many others. Soon we were rounding the Cape, where many ships went into Cape Town; but we sailed on into Durban, reaching it on 13 February.

Although South Africa was with us in the war, Durban was just as in peacetime, or so it seemed to us. The hospitality we received there was unforgettable – the one snag was the enormous humidity. We were driven around, often by young ladies, and shown the lovely scenery nearby; were taken to the races, homes or hotels for food, and we swam in the ocean. I earned a small fee for a 15 minute radio broadcast with Marine Jack Llewellyn, currently the best known British jazz guitarist. One evening when I was on duty I saw a patient with ocular skew deviation – alcoholic of course. He was quite all right next morning. After our four days in Durban we sailed north to stop for one day in Aden. Then we sailed up the Red Sea to dock at Suez on 8 March 1942. Before disembarking I was informed that I was medical officer to 227 Squadron, but that was all I was told.

After disembarking, the RAF doctors reported to the PMO at HQME in Cairo. Had I expected words like "Astley, thank God you are here!" I would have been disappointed. What I got was to be told to go away for a few days whilst they found out what I was supposed to be doing. I put up at a poorish hotel and trudged around Cairo, and in the process had my wallet stolen. So when I returned to HQME it was for a loan first and instructions second – I got both and I was sent to a large maintenance unit in the canal zone where I met up with 350 men, the ground staff for 227 Squadron, which was yet to form. To make matters worse there was only one admin officer and he was promptly posted, leaving me holding the fort as acting CO. This went on for about 10 days; we were under canvas and the winds were blowing gales each day – everything was covered in sand. So I gave the troops lectures in hygiene, organised football and a concert party, and even conducted a pay parade. Then another officer turned up, elderly and full of grumbles, which increased as the weeks passed by. We had hung around for the best part of two months when at last transport began to arrive and we began to cheer up until, to my horror, we received two water carts. We were routed to a desert airfield, Geniaclis, just near to the western edge of the Nile Delta – one side a vine area run by a Greek (wine a shilling per bottle) and just sand to the west. We set ourselves up as best we could and other officers began to arrive. Water was high priority and my medical corporal, a real bright lad and clearly destined to do well in life, suggested that all we need do was to take the two water carts just five miles along a desert track and fill them up from a tap where the water supply was known to be safe, and this procedure worked very well.

High spirits

More disappointments lay ahead, however; although a few Beaufighters and crews had arrived we were never fully established. One evening, shortly after I had seen my first scorpion hiding in a corner of our mess, we got a signal instructing all the ground staff to proceed to Aqir in Palestine where we would form up with a squadron of heavy bombers, Halifaxes, shortly flying out from the UK, whilst our few Beaufighters and crews would join another such unit. The men took this with good humour – we had only

11

been five weeks at Geniaclis and I could sense some pride and esprit de corps developing. On 25 June we were all packed up and we went by road to Kantara to cross the canal by ferry. This procedure took some time as there were units of the Ninth Army moving the other way to support the Eighth Army at Alamein. I remember the joke got around that the German spotter planes would not know whether the British were advancing or retreating. After we crossed most of the men went by train, though there was a further delay as the engine blew up, but eventually a replacement arrived and we reached Aqir about 3 am, and rather than pitch tents in the darkness we fell asleep on the grass surrounding the runway. Next morning dozens reported sick with insect and other bites, probably due to centipedes in this area; they were nasty looking objects, six or more inches long and they moved a serpiginous course like a train. The Halifaxes soon arrived and we were soon on good terms with the aircrews, though we poked fun at them when they declared they were in the middle east for 16 days only – we thought we knew better, and so it proved.

In the time we had been at Geniaclis the officers' and men's messes had accumulated both money and stock, by which I mean booze, and permission was requested of our new CO, and granted, that we have a party and dance, there being no blackout in Palestine. I was declared to be entertainments officer and given the task of organising this affair – and what a shambles it turned out. I hired a hall in the small town nearby, a six piece band, extra stocks of drink from the NAAFI, and QA nurses from two army hospitals nearby, 12 and 23 at Sarafand. I also recruited lots of Palestinian ATS females. The mistake was to allow other ranks to have spirits as well as beer, and to open the bars for 15 minutes before the ladies arrived. By the time they did arrive there were many drunken airmen around, singing and shouting, fighting and falling, and the broken glass on the floor made dancing hazardous. I had to close the whole thing down and have the ladies taken home; the party had not lasted longer than about an hour, and next day I was going around making apologies to matrons and others, explaining that our men were really suffering from desert fatigue – I could think of nothing better to say, remembering that my name was on every ticket.

It was at Aqir, where I now had a hutted bedroom, that I saw the biggest spider ever, a large hairy giant on my bedroom wall just above my bed. It was cunning, too, for as I moved one end of my bed it moved the other way. I picked up a cricket bat I happened to have in my room, pulled the whole bed away from the wall, took careful aim, and hit it first time; it fell to the floor and I crushed it with my boot ... then I could sleep. But we were to be in this pleasant countryside only a few weeks and on 13 August we moved back to Fayid in the canal zone where a new RAF runway and station had been completed. The war news was good and at Fayid we could see for ourselves evidence of the huge build up from the many trains passing close by going north from Suez stacked with guns, tanks, and other hardware. I was appointed mess president and soon afterwards promoted to squadron leader – clearly the authorities had not yet heard about our dance at Aqir. I remember we had a special RAF Liberator unit, and these lads flew over Yugoslavia nightly dropping agents; it was all very secret, though everyone knew of course. The participants were brought to a special room, and we had to provide them with a hot dinner, yet these men were not supposed to be seen by anyone. I cannot recall any aircraft going missing on these missions, which took 14 hours' flying time. At Fayid we had important visitors, first the AOCME Tedder, then later Lord Trenchard ("Boom"), our founder, a marvellous old man who gave us a splendidly stirring address. The big push at Alamein began on 24 October and all aircrews were flying several missions a day, and giving blood for our transfusion campaign as well. It was all very exciting to realise that here was the turning point in the war – surely this time it must be right.

On the move again

We moved forward again on 9 November to a desert airfield 40 kilometres northwest of Cairo, and it was here I had the only taste of professional trouble I ever encountered in the air force. I had sent a 50 year old officer into the RAF Hospital in Cairo for a check up; he was dyspnoeic and I thought it might be cardiac and that he was probably not fit to move further into the western desert. Our new CO, whom I regarded as an erratic and paranoid character, ordered me to have this officer discharged from hospital and brought back to our unit. I refused to do this, explained why, but to no avail. Although I had a rule never to ask for nor to refuse a posting, I got into my ambulance and drove past the pyramids down into HQME in Cairo that evening and saw the duty officer for medical personnel. I told him my story and I asked for a posting ... anywhere. In a week I was posted to RAF Takali, Malta, retaining my rank. Because of my cabin trunk I opted to go by sea and on 28 December I sailed from Alexandria on HMS *Exmoor*, with three other destroyers escorting one oil tanker and one merchant ship for Malta. The journey was full of interest and luckily we had pretty good air cover, the desert army having captured Benghazi and its airfield. I slept in the wardroom, and was allowed on the bridge to listen to the Asdic probing the depths. We had no alcohol, not even on New Year's Eve, and we sailed into Grand Harbour on 2 January with cheering crowds lining the ramparts.

Takali airstrip was below Rabat and Mdina towards the centre of the island. The mess was in a large house in Mdina where from the roof terrace there was a wonderful view, and where I soon had a nice bedroom with a tiled bathroom, though no hot water. We had a medical emergency unit carved into the quarry near the airstrip, and a separate sick quarters in Rabat with beds. Malta was green at this time, but very depressing with all shops boarded up and signs of bomb damage everywhere. Our diet was poor, corned beef alternating with pilchards, powdered milk and potatoes, and no fruit or vegetables. There was an epidemic of polio, and 90% of the population had scabies. Some of the RAF giants had left, one way or another, but some were still there, and I shared the bedroom with Wing Commander Buchanan, a remarkable young man with some 25 enemy scalps to his credit. He had greatly exceeded his flying hours and should have been grounded but refused. He was disdainful of aircrew who had lost confidence and tried to get out of flying, nor was it RAF policy to make this easy for them. He was eventually lost in his Beaufighter over Greece, but I cannot forget his golden hair, tiny moustache, his courage, and his fondness for the ladies.

Meeting Monty

Tunis fell on 13 May and with it the north African campaign ended. This was the signal for the Malta build up and by the end of June Malta's harbours were packed with carriers, battleships, and all kinds of naval craft including landing craft; the airfields now housed 28 squadrons of RAF, and a lot of the Eighth Army were spread about 30 camps – what an exciting time this was. Six more doctors arrived at our mess with a Spitfire wing, making nine in all for about 2000 personnel – medical overmanning? We were in turn visited by Portal, Tedder, Sholto Douglas; later the DGMS Whittingham, and then His Majesty King George on 20 June. Finally on 4 July came General Montgomery, and I was privileged to be invited to our underground HQ at Takali to meet him with the squadron commanders. I thought Monty was very impressive indeed, sharp eyed and inquisitive. He shook me by the hand and asked about health and morale, and the others he asked how far the Spits could fly with and without extra fuel tanks, and he wanted Kitty bombers. No one mentioned Sicily at that meeting, but the invasion began five days later on 9 July and to my surprise I went with the Spitfire wing from Takali on 16 July. This happened through an unhappy incident, as on 10 July the senior doctor to the wing was arrested on a security matter and was flown to Tripoli for court martial. On 12 July his body was picked out of the sea at Tripoli. Thus I was attached to take his place for the time being. We sailed on an infantry landing craft from Valetta in moonlight and a calm sea. I was not feeling well and could not eat anything all that day; when I was offered pilchards on the journey I vomited. We entered Syracuse harbour at dawn, and in intense heat awaited our transport, then moved in convoy along the coast road north to Augusta. I vomited and wondered if it was the quinine or simply neurosis. Next morning, after a poor night in a bivouac, I shaved and saw that my conjunctivae had turned yellow. I was flown by air ambulance to 90 General Hospital in Malta, to the surprise of many of the staff whom I knew there. After a week or so the recovery began, and I went to rest camp at St Paul's Bay on 7 August. Noel Coward appeared one day and entertained us on his own with stories (rude) and songs – we all roared when we heard for the first time his song "Don't let's be beastly to the Germans".

On 13 August I returned to my old job at Takali, but it seemed empty and quiet now, as indeed the real war had passed Malta by and the excitement had gone. In a sense too, the war was over for me. I was moved to Luqa, and I stayed on Malta until I was repatriated in December 1944. During that year Malta slowly returned to a normal life with goods and food now plentiful, but there was lots to be done. On my return to the UK I was posted to a Lancaster bomber station at Waddington in Lincolnshire after marrying the girl who had refused me three years before – she is still with me. I must have been at a party in the officers' mess at Waddington on VE Day, but I cannot remember it at all, and no prizes for guessing the reason. Whatever was the reason, I cannot remember VJ Day either – it must be global amnesia. The RAF finally freed me on 23 January 1946 after five and a half happy years.

Plenty to do

JOSEPHINE BARNES

In August 1939 we spent a family holiday in France. We stayed in a tiny village on the Lake of Annecy. So remote was it that we missed the radio announcement advising British residents to return home, but return we did in great discomfort in crowded trains.

A week later, on that Sunday morning, we heard Chamberlain's announcement telling us that we were at war with Germany. It had begun, the war we had all feared and anticipated since Hitler had taken control of Germany, invaded Austria and Czechoslovakia, and, finally, Poland. It was to be a long, hard, and dark road to 8 May 1945 when the war in Europe came to an end.

I spent most of the war years in London, apart from one year in Oxford. After so long the memories are somewhat blurred, but the main impressions remain. Outstanding was the amazing spirit of the people of London, cheerful often amid the smoking ruins of their homes in the blitz and during the flying bomb raids. On the whole they preferred to be underground during air raids. This meant climbing over the sleeping bodies in the tube stations on the way home in the evening.

Of course there were many inconveniences. There was the blackout, and driving with little light was sometimes hair raising, especially if one was looking for a house where there was an obstetric emergency. But I remember little mugging or robbery – we hadn't much worth stealing. There was food rationing, which everyone accepted, and though at times we were hungry it did us little harm. In fact the rationing became more stringent after the war was over. Clothes were rationed and so we became shabbier as time went on. Some people made dresses from curtain material until that was rationed too. Holidays were few and short – there was not enough staff in the hospitals for us to be spared for long.

Opportunity for women

In the hospitals there was plenty of work to be done: babies were born, women came with gynaecological problems, the medical students had to be taught, and casualty departments were busy especially after air raids. The evacuees of the early days of the war slowly drifted back to London so that all hospital departments were busy. At University College Hospital, where I worked for a large part of the war, the men were called up and disappeared one by one. Each medical student was allowed one six month house job before being called up. This meant that women doctors did a good deal of the work, an opportunity many of us relished.

In spite of the blackout all was not gloom. The theatres and the opera were open and there were promenade concerts at the dear old Queen's Hall, until that was bombed, and then at the Albert Hall. Myra Hess's lunchtime concerts at the National Gallery were also popular. There were many restaurants open. The rule was that no meal must cost more than 5 shillings – unless there was dancing, in which case it could be 7/6.

After D Day – 6 June 1944 – it at last began to seem that the end might be in sight. Most of us had husbands, brothers, and friends involved in that great enterprise, and the desperate battles, and at times the slow progress, were anxiously watched. The flying bombs and the V2 rockets began and these made life very unpleasant for a while. I happened to have a few days off in Essex after a minor illness and watched the gliders going over on their way to Arnhem. Gradually the armies progressed towards Germany and the air raids ceased, to our great relief. Then at last the Germans surrendered and it was VE Day.

Euphoria and after

My recollections of that day are reasonably vivid. I must have done a day's work in London and then gone home to Barnet where we were living with my parents and our young daughter. In the evening – my husband was home on leave – we went back to London. Luckily we didn't take the small car we had been lent but went by tube.

London had gone mad! Trafalgar Square was packed with a happy crowd; but the crowd became more and more excited. Cars were overturned and some set on fire – justification for travelling by a safer method. The crowd surged to Buckingham Palace where the King and Queen, with Princess Elizabeth and Princess Margaret, appeared on the balcony with Winston Churchill, and the crowds cheered and cheered and would not let them go. The lights went up for the first time in almost six years. We repaired to the Junior Carlton Club, then in St James's Square but overlooking Pall Mall. For the first and last time I was allowed into the hallowed all male part of the club. The crowds surged along Pall Mall on the way to the palace. The only thing missing was fireworks, not permitted in wartime.

After the euphoria of VE Day there was the long climb back to normality. Churchill lost the election and was replaced by Clement Attlee. There were still relatives and friends fighting the Japanese and in prison in Singapore and Malaysia. Roosevelt had died and been replaced by Harry Truman. The Russians had spread out over eastern Europe.

Then came the dropping of the atomic bombs on Japan and the Japanese surrender. VJ Day, 15 August, was a comparatively quiet occasion, almost an anticlimax after the excitements of VE Day. Demobilisation had not yet got under way and the men were still in the services so that work in London continued in the same hectic way.

On VJ Day I went with a friend to the theatre. I cannot remember what the play was but I do remember the arrival of Mr and Mrs Churchill with their daughter Mary, and the tremendous ovation they received.

The war was really over.

Almost like any other day

R I S BAYLISS

VE Day started, and almost finished, like any other day. Four years of war, spent in a teaching hospital, had brought a restricted, even rigid, pattern to life. To many, I suspect, the lack of ability to make personal decisions, the tight rationing system, the fixed pay, the immediacy of survival, the corporate unselfseeking commitment had dulled our reactions. We did not apply for medical jobs, we were directed. Whether we remained at hospital or were drafted was not of our choosing. The nation became more egalitarian, more classless. In retrospect I think we were stultified. Perhaps this was because of Churchill's remarkable leadership, and perhaps also because of the information given to us by the press and the BBC. Very rarely did I suspect that we were being subjected to "propaganda". It says much for the "honesty" of the heavily controlled media that we believed implicitly what we were told. And in general I think that what we were told was true. We accepted the bad news of disasters with the good news of our victories. Every now and then something was reported that didn't ring quite true, and I would resolve to find out after the war what the real truth was. I never have, because the water has long since passed under the bridge.

Working at St Thomas's was a total commitment. There was no off duty, no free weekends, seldom an hour in the day when one could slip more than 50 yards away from the hospital to buy the much needed but usually unobtainable new safety razor blade. You simply stayed in the hospital and worked. In retrospect this brought amazing clinical experience, but at some price to one's general education. It may explain my later difficulty in accepting units of medical time and three in one rotas.

Endless hours

I've forgotten how often, according to the official record, the hospital was hit by bombs. Seventy six is the number that comes to mind but I cannot vouch for its accuracy. The first fell when Robert Donat was making a film in an unused part of the hospital. Some physiotherapists sleeping in the block adjacent to Westminster Bridge were trapped under the rubble. The salvage corps rescued them by jacking up the beams that compressed their bodies. They were alive when extricated; one died shortly afterwards. At that time we knew nothing of the pathology of crush injuries and, if I remember rightly, it was Eric Bywaters (later to be a colleague and professor of rheumatology at the Royal Postgraduate Medical School) who taught us about the renal damage caused by myoglobin. Nor will I forget the morning when a V1 made a direct hit on a double decker bus filled with city gents outside Waterloo Station. Our casualty department looked like Gettysburg. My job was to sort the wheat from the tares, a procedure later to be given the scientific appellation "triage". When I came to anaesthetise (with Pentothal, nitrous oxide, ether, and oxygen from an old Boyle's apparatus) one of the patients selected for early surgery in the bowels of the hospital, it seemed to me that she was in remarkably good shape for someone with a compound fracture of the right femur. I said to my surgical registrar colleague (Paddy Kelly, later an eminent urologist) that I thought we should have an x ray done before he proceeded further. The x ray, taken in the theatre and delaying procedures badly, showed that the secretary bird's femur was intact. She was lucky not to have lost her leg. What was sticking out of her thigh was a piece of someone else's femur, and Paddy removed this, cleaned the wound, sprinkled in some sulphonamide powder, and left it at that.

We worked endless hours. There were casualties from the bombing; there were "ordinary" patients. These varied from the sublime to the ridiculous. I think I was a casualty officer, qualified for two weeks, when a young girl came in complaining that she had something wrong with her "love box". This was beyond my expertise and I called in the selfsame Paddy Kelly who had been qualified all of two years. Tactfully I stood on the other side of the screen as he examined her. I remember hearing him say, in a cheerful and encouraging tone, "Not only a love box, dear, but a letter box!"

We knew, before VE Day, that the war in Europe was going to end soon. This realisation brought relief, but some apprehension. The apprehension was largely based on the continuing war in the Pacific. Because of the geography this seemed likely to last nearly as long as the European war had done. We had absolutely no inkling of the development of nuclear fission, or that two atom bombs would fall on Japan and bring a precipitate end to hostilities. Consciously or subconsciously we were also fearful of a change, a major change, in our lives. No longer would we be directed by the governmental decisions which we had placidly accepted for so long. For many people the resumption of a free life with the ability to make free decisions led to anxiety. Heretofore what we did and where we did it was dictated from on high. Our pay, which did not enter our thinking, was fixed. What we could spend on food was also fixed. The economy was as immutable as one presumes it is today under a communist regime. But because of our common purpose this was comfortably accepted.

Too busy to notice

VE Day started as just another day. Peace in Europe would bring an end to the V2 missiles that fell on London. V2s were unacceptable – and unnerving. They came in a trajectory which gave no audible warning, and hence the noise of their explosion occurred several seconds after they had wrought their devastation. V1s were much more "fair". You could hear them coming and you could hear when the propelling rocket ran out of fuel. With good binaural hearing you could make a reasonable guess as to where it was going to land. On the first night that V1 missiles were launched in substantial numbers, I sat on a parapet on the roof of St Thomas's with a porter who had served in the RAMC in World War I. We watched these jet propelled aeroplanes, as I thought they were, approaching London from the south east; we saw the jet flame cease and then the "aeroplane" dive down, followed by the inevitable explosion. The anti-aircraft guns were firing furiously. I turned to Johnson and said, "The Ack-ack are doing unbelievably well tonight". Johnson shook his head in polite disagreement. "I think they are 'itler's secret weapon," he said. With youthful pomposity I stood up. "Johnson," I said. "Rubbish. I don't want to hear any more of that sort of talk." Not until the morning papers arrived did I learn with shame that indeed Hitler had launched his first secret weapon.

During those years at St Thomas's Hospital we saw little daylight. All the windows had been bricked up; the heart of the hospital (the operating theatres and the canteen) were in the basement; our lives were spent in perpetual electric light.

The news of the German surrender passed almost unnoticed as we worked on the wards and coped with outpatients. We were but an oasis in London. Beds had to be cleared for the next emergency and patients were transferred as soon as possible on stretchers in specially adapted Green Line buses to Guildford and Godalming. One such patient was a Cypriot waiter. He had come to casualty with some lumps on his nose and face. The casualty officer, qualified one week, had examined him and sent the notes up to me for further action. As resident assistant physician I had remarkable responsibility for my 24 years. When the notes arrived I was having tea with my chief, Sir Maurice Cassidy, and laughingly showed him the notes. "The casualty officer has diagnosed leprosy," I said disparagingly. "Let's go and look," suggested Sir Maurice. Sure enough there was the first case of leprosy that I (or he) had ever seen. Dr Joseph Bamforth, our pathologist, had already found the Hansen bacillus in a nasal swab. The patient had to be transferred for treatment to a sector hospital and was put on a Green Line ambulance bus to go to Guildford. A few hours later a telephone call from Warren Road (later St Luke's) Hospital complained bitterly that I had infected the bus, the other patients in it, and the entire hospital. I tried to point out that the biblical contagiousness of leprosy was entirely wrong but Guildford was not prepared to accept my non-expert opinion. How many cases of leprosy had I seen? The matter would be reported to higher authority. An hour later I had a telephone call from the eminent leprosy adviser to the Ministry of Health, and our Cypriot was accepted with equanimity.

Thus we worked throughout the day, and on similar days I saw as many as 120 patients. The great event occurring across the Channel passed almost unnoticed until 5 o'clock in the evening. Then an old girl friend rang. We must celebrate. She was friendly with a Canadian brigadier who had brought over a gramophone record of *Oklahoma*, the first of the new great American musicals. Would I come round and join them for dinner? I would. Thus that night a Canadian staff car with driver, the Canadian brigadier, and the ex-girl friend and I drove from St Thomas's through the thronging crowds to Leicester Square. The "400" was the most respectable of night clubs but one I could ill afford on a registrar's salary. The three of us sat there in the dim light drinking a legally "prepurchased" bottle of Scotch and danced to Tim Clayton and his band playing the tunes of *Oklahoma* until one in the morning when I walked up the ramp to the entrance of the casualty department and St Thomas's Hospital.

*   *   *

Elston Grey-Turner and I had been good friends at Cambridge. He had been chairman of the Cambridge University Medical Society and I had been one of his committee members. With the help of his influential father he produced many notable lecturers for the Medical Society. As so often happens when Cambridge graduates go to different teaching hospitals, I had lost touch with him but heard he had fractured a bone in his foot while drilling recruits in north Africa. We laughed, because this was typical of Elston's enthusiasm. This enthusiasm I was to admire even more when many years later we served together on the board of Private Patients Plan. I still have a photograph of the Cambridge Medical Society Committee in 1936. Elston's image remains unchanged, and just as respected and loved.

A bad memory of something good

DOUGLAS BLACK

I am, of course, delighted and honoured to have been asked to contribute a piece to a memorial volume for Elston Grey-Turner, whom I adored and respected in equal measure. And I shall try to overcome two difficulties, one general and the other more particular. The general one is that, by chance, my particular line of military service in the RAMC, consisting as it did at the relevant time of close attention to the stools of military personnel suffering from sprue, would not have made an instant appeal to Elston's strong sense of military duty. The second, more particular, difficulty in contributing to a volume of recollections of VE Day is that I honestly can't remember what I was up to on that particular occasion. But perhaps I can serve as some kind of lowly control by trying to give an impression of what it was like to be a "support troop" and, as a result of that posting, to be much more of a spectator than many civilians in the front line, facing V1s and V2s.

Let me begin by trying to explain to those who were then in Europe, and who may be amazed that anyone could fail to recall such a milestone as VE Day must have been to them, how it could happen that it made comparatively little impact on people in other continents, for I was certainly not unique in my reaction.

View from India

We had indeed been intensely interested in the long awaited D Day, and in the overcoming of the Ardennes crisis in the 1944–5 winter; but for weeks before it actually came the end of the European war had been clearly in sight, and from our distance the actual day of surrender was something of a foregone conclusion. We remained conscious of the formidable enemy still active in the east, and of course we knew nothing of the doom that was being prepared for Hiroshima (possibly defensible under the stress of war, against a determined and ruthless enemy) and for Nagasaki (indefensible under any circumstances, I believe, given the impact of the first bomb). I confess with shame that the news of Hiroshima was received with some tincture of relief by those who had been overseas for several years, in that it shortened the likely duration of the conflict. By the time of the second bomb, some days later, we had learned more of the scale of destruction, and were beginning to have a dim suspicion of the reign of terror which might lie ahead.

Like the great majority of people in all ages, or at least the majority of those who know where their next meal is coming from, we were more concerned with our personal duties and recreations than with the secular turmoil around us. To be more personal, I was doing interesting work with reasonably good facilities, and with excellent and congenial colleagues. I don't know the meaning of a "good" war – to me, all wars are bad, even if, like the war of 1939–45, they are made inevitable by wickedness or carelessness in high places – but we had a comfortable war, at least during the particular phase of it that I spent in Poona, a place which was remarkable only in the truth of the unlikely seeming anecdotes told about it. For example, it is direct experience which allows me to recall that when Earl J King came out to visit our laboratory he was debarred from the dining room of the Poona Club, since he had not brought a dinner jacket with him (they were not being much worn at the time, at home). Of course the kindly Indian servants did not let him starve – they gave him his dinner outside on the lawn, behind a screen so that he was not visible from the dining room. (Paul Fourman and I rescued him the following day, and he was from then on a splendid companion in the hospital mess.)

There was an element of remoteness in India, which lessened the tangibility of even the most dramatic events. The media of information also lacked a certain sophistication. For example, there was a newspaper called the *Daily Kal*, which sounds innocent enough, until you discover that the Urdu word "kal" can mean either "yesterday" or "tomorrow". This puts even crisp expressions of intent like "mañana" into the shade.

Right dress

I have a recollection that the central military pathology laboratory did have a victory parade, I think only one, in the courtyard; but I don't recall whether it was for VE Day or VJ Day. As a group, we were inclined to play the rules according to the game rather than the other way round; but our colonel, a fine man, was a regular and liked to do the right thing. I fear that at times we may have been something of a trial to him. On one occasion, when we were using bunsen burners in the summer heat, Paul and I had taken off our bush shirts. The colonel happened to come in and remonstrated with us, on the basis that if, say, a corporal happened to come in with a specimen, he might not recognise that we were officers (and possibly favour us with some language unfit for delicate ears). Paul's offer to have crowns tattooed on our shoulders was not accepted – and now that I know more about tattooing I am glad.

*   *   *

Ah well, perhaps we were young and careless; and of course VE Day was notable, though perhaps more as a symbol than as an event in its own right. It was thoroughly selfish of us not to perceive more clearly the relief for those who had been fighting up to that day – but for those at home the front line war had already ended with the capture of the V2 sites. And I think I have been honest, and not too unfair, in suggesting that for us temporary sahibs the day may have been little more eventful than Conan Doyle's dog's failure to bark in the night.

Lessons in surgery, geography, and much else

GUY BLACKBURN

Life in a field surgical unit – in which I had been serving since July 1944, and previously in another unit of the same type with the First Army in north Africa – suddenly reverted to the orthodox, surgically speaking, with the victory in Europe in May 1945. From then on there were, happily, no more battle casualties but surgical work of a less urgent variety, with the tempo of evacuation much less pressing and the problems of repatriation of large numbers of enemy casualties added to those of the homeward journey of our own wounded, many for further surgical treatment at base hospitals in the UK.

The final phase

The advance through northen Italy from Forli in November 1944 to Russi and Lugo in April 1945 had contrasted with easier days on the Adriatic coast – with incomparable beaches such as Rimini and Riccione – the previous summer, and the last of our battle casualties were dealt with in Quartesana and Copparo before we moved across the border into Austria. In all 237 cases were treated between September 1944 and May 1945, and it was noteworthy that they included a higher proportion of prisoners of war than heretofore, as well as civilians and partisans. Arriving in Klagenfurt on VE Day the unit cooperated with a field dressing station in taking over a large military hospital, housing a large number of enemy wounded and some prisoners of war. Many of these were British, who spoke highly of the care they had received from the German army medical services – by that time operating under difficult conditions, with supplies of drugs and equipment rapidly diminishing and woefully inadequate in many respects.

The long haul up the east coast of Italy, the battle for the Po

Valley in particular, and the adverse weather conditions in the mountains in winter had taught us a new set of lessons to add to experience in Algeria and Tunisia, where the winter of 1942 had likewise been severe, but the summer of 1943 very hot indeed – particularly in tented accommodation before the fall of Tunis in May of that year. Time had begun to march more rapidly when my batman greeted me on 6 June 1944 with the opening gambit of, "Nice morning for an invasion, sir". It would be hard to exaggerate the effect on morale which the BBC news and the voice of the Prime Minister in particular had on us all, notably when the fall of the Chancellery in Berlin ultimately became inevitable: and the final news of victory in Europe on 8 May produced a measure of euphoria, almost in disbelief. This inevitably was expressed in riotous celebration, accompanied by Austrian beer and wine in incredible quantities – I had seen nothing like it since the fall of Tunis, when wine actually ran down the gutters in the streets.

The sequel to this extravaganza in 1945 varied from unit to unit, my own colleagues in the field surgical unit suddenly experiencing a desire to catch horses (there were so many free) and ride them, albeit without any previous riding experience. The subsequent crop of fractures of the pelvis in CMF, with and without complications, produced surgical problems of a new variety.

But VE Day itself was the occasion of a tumultuous welcome from the civilian population, and protracted rejoicing. This was coupled with an intense thankfulness among us that London and our cities in the British Isles were no longer the targets for "doodlebugs" and "buzz bombs", of which we had no personal experience. High explosive aerial bombing and landmines were familiar to us from the days before we left the UK but later variations of aerial attack – like pilotless planes and guided missiles – were largely an unknown quantity. It was then a marvellous relief to know that the banshee wailing of sirens would no longer harbinger attacks on civilian targets, indeed on our families and friends in civil life, whose lot we all knew had often been harder to bear than our own. Demobilisation would occur at a rate inversely proportional to mobilisation but the knowledge that it was appreciably nearer now made the war in the east the only obstacle.

The overall experience

It is well known that the prototype of the field surgical unit was conceived in the western desert in 1941–2 and 12 units of a new type accompanied the First Army in the north African invasion. The basic structure of a surgeon and anaesthetist with one NCO and five RAMC other ranks meant that the unit was not autonomous and depended on a field ambulance, field dressing station, or casualty clearing station for rations and maintenance. Three RASC personnel looked after the transport (a staff car and two three ton lorries), and the possession of tentage and, particularly, 12 beds proved invaluable. These enabled wounded men – especially with abdominal or thoracic wounds – to be held for as much as 7–10 days before evacuation to a lower echelon. It had a significant effect on the attendant morbidity and mortality.

Originally the FSUs were attached to field ambulances or casualty clearing stations in north Africa, but it was gradually realised that a field dressing station or casualty clearing station were really the most suitable parent units. The paramount importance of nursing in these units by officers of the Queen Alexandra Military Nursing Service had to be seen to be believed. This is not to decry the work of male nursing orderlies in the RAMC in the earlier phases of the campaign, but trained female nurses were what the patients expected in civil life and they certainly responded very quickly as soon as their counterparts arrived to take care of them in war.

It is difficult to appraise the impression made on us by the wide variety of military patients who came under our care, not to mention the civilians – Arabs and Italians in particular – and of course German prisoners of war. All these provided their separate challenges and the adaptability of the RAMC personnel was a never failing source of surprise. The language difficulty somehow never provided an insuperable barrier, and common denominators like cigarettes and eggs rapidly became almost international currency.

I would find it hard to exaggerate the enormous contribution in triage and resuscitation made by field transfusion units, and nothing contributed more to the salvage and recovery rate than the availability of blood, once this became a reality. The era of antibiotics was only just dawning but in powder form it was perhaps the greatest factor in the success of delayed primary closure of wounds in the last two years of the war. Many lessons were learnt by surgeons in the field in the hard school of surgical endeavour, and problems such as gas gangrene were very quickly

30

appreciated and put in perspective, with practical experience virtually the only worthwhile qualification in dealing with this otherwise frightening complication. The management of patients in a manner designed to secure their earliest evacuation quickly became familiar with practice, an excellent example being the "Tobruk" plaster for fractures of the femur.

It remained a source of wonder and admiration that nursing orderlies from all walks of life – an assortment from Lancashire, Yorkshire, Warwickshire, Devon, and London in one unit – quickly became an integrated and basically happy team, with the proverbial genius of the British soldier for improvisation and traditional imperturbability in face of apparently overwhelming odds. Tented accommodation in African countries and all manner of buildings in the Italian theatre seemed to come alike, and the rapidity with which a primus stove and mug of "char" would appear at unlikely moments defied all ordinary laws of probability.

Respite from war

The lessons in geography, ethnic considerations, and cooperation with a legion of differing racial creeds were unique – as only war would provide on this scale. And as victory dawned, and at last became a reality, it was a privilege to reflect that every man would savour the experience in retrospect and count himself lucky to have had the opportunity and to have survived.

The Austrian lakes and countryside promised a respite from war at last and in the event we were not to be disappointed.

Who better deserved it, in my opinion, than these men, who had adapted themselves so splendidly to support their comrades in arms in the field? They typified the words of Winston Churchill: "The nation had the lion's heart" and the lion had prevailed at last.

Reserved occupation

D E BOLT

Curiously, I have few recollections of VE Day. I remember that I was on duty as fracture house surgeon at Bristol Royal Infirmary, although still some months short of qualification. During the last year of the war doctors were allowed only three months after qualification for house jobs before being called up for duty in the armed forces, so that students spent much of their final year filling gaps in the resident staff. I remember that from the windows of the residents' quarters at the BRI one could hear the distant roar of an assembled multitude in the tramway centre, but, as casualty was inevitably rather busy, the celebration passed me by. Indeed, as medical students were in a "reserved occupation" and subject to call up only on qualification, VE Day did not bring, for me, the sudden release from personal danger which demanded noisy or alcoholic celebration.

Of course, there had been the air raids which allowed us, in our rather embarrassingly favoured situation, the feeling of taking some share in the dangers which less fortunate people accepted constantly. We were all active in some aspect of civil defence, whether in mobile first aid units (as I was), fire watching, or, in the clinical years, helping to deal with casualties as they arrived at the hospital. Fire watching entailed patrolling the roof of the hospital buildings, armed with buckets of sand and long handled shovels, or buckets of water and stirrup pumps, ready to deal with incendiary bombs as soon as they landed and before their intense magnesium fires could start a serious conflagration. It was very valuable work and many buildings, including the ancient church of St Mary Redcliffe in Bristol, survived the blitz because of prompt work by fire watchers; but it was not without its hazards and those engaged in it could feel quite remarkably exposed, walking a high roof to the accompaniment of the strangely hostile drone of bombers' engines, the scream of falling bombs and the crump of anti-aircraft guns; and with a wide view of the city, barrage balloons silhouetted against the unearthly glow of fires already out of control, and the whole scene brilliantly illuminated by wandering searchlights and the cold light of a "bombers' moon". Even after the period of almost nightly raids was over, immediately available fire watchers remained essential and, for many medical students, such duties became a welcome pattern of life. Provided with a bed, supper, and breakfast, and a small nightly payment, many became permanently resident in the evacuated upper floors of the hospitals, a valuable arrangement in the days before student grants.

Silent endurance

Looking back now on the period when air raids were very frequent I am mainly impressed by the extraordinary endurance of the ordinary citizens. They sat out the raids, night after weary night, in air raid shelters or crouched under the stairs of their houses, cuddling children or terrified pets, listening to the inferno outside and, for the sake of those about them, assuming a jauntiness which belied their true anxieties. There was a widespread, and almost certainly inaccurate, belief that you would not hear the whistle of the bomb which hit you, which allowed people to call reassurance to each other however near the scream of the bomb might sound, forgetting that falling masonry was as powerful a killer as a direct hit. To listen, in total impotence, to the approaching explosions of a stick of bombs, trying uselessly to gauge from the apparent distance between the fourth and fifth whether the still awaited sixth would fall on you, was not something that people could reasonably be expected to endure, although they did so regularly for endless months. Those of us with something to do during air raids were protected from this kind of experience and, at the time, gave little thought to the silent endurance of the ordinary citizen.

My closest personal contact with the war came about the time of D Day. Students in their second clinical year were asked to volunteer for some nationally important task and, while no overt mention was made of the impending invasion of Europe, the purpose was evident to us all. With a close friend from my year I was attached to an ambulance train, improvised from a passenger coach and dining car, which provided living quarters, and a series of parcel vans with racks for stretchers, which were the wards. It was manned by a number of orderlies, ourselves, and an elderly and very charming psychiatrist, who had overall charge. On a specified day we joined the train in a siding near Bristol and travelled to Southampton, where we were parked in the dock area. There we sat for about a week, watching the assembly of a major part of the invasion force.

Convoys of lorries arrived bringing troops to the vast barbed wire enclosures in the dock area, whence, in due course, they embarked in a variety of vessels such as large tank landing craft, smaller troop carriers, and major ships, from which they would be carried to the beaches in smaller landing craft unsuitable for the Channel crossing fully loaded. Tanks, troop carriers, lorries, and huge quantities of military stores were similarly loaded and, as each vessel completed its complement of men and equipment, it moved out into the Solent to await the order to go. Among the transport ships, numerous naval craft came and went incessantly, occasionally shouting imperiously by loud hailer at any vessel in danger of missing its place in the predetermined queue. Our stay was enlivened by the occasional "doodle bug", which caused no anxiety if its engine was still running when overhead, but which made a search for cover urgent if the engine died before reaching you. By the afternoon of 5 June the activity on the docks was noticably diminishing and, as darkness fell, the ships we could see at anchor, in response to the quick flickering of signal lamps from the escorting warships, quietly slipped away.

Officers and men

The morning of 6 June seemed strangely quiet on Southampton docks, in comparison with the frenzied activity of the previous days, but late in the evening a Southern Railway schools class locomotive appeared out of the darkness and moved us to the dockside. Towards midnight the first of many hospital ships came in and, in a short time, we were loading our first casualties. They were sorted at the gangway by a RAMC colonel, in other times a surgeon at the Royal Victoria Hospital at Belfast, who decided on those for local hospitalisation and those suitable to carry to one of the sector hospitals, just south of London. The troops we carried were all commandos or paratroops who had been responsible for preparing the way for the major landings on the Normandy beaches and we began with a bad mistake which, as we were only civilians, they overlooked. We had been instructed that we should have separate "wards" for officers and other ranks and, indeed, later on we had such an arrangement; but it was rapidly made clear to us that these closely knit groups of men were not going to be separated on that basis. I was, rather primly, surprised to hear officers addressed by their Christian names by their men and it was my first lesson in how little real authority has to do with the word "Sir". The less seriously wounded were greatly concerned for the more serious casualties – "Will he be all right, Doc?" – to which a medical student's response could only be uninformed reassurance. They were endlessly talkative, endlessly anxious for news we did not possess and, in fact, behaved as men will, unwinding after great danger with the knowledge that their roles in the enterprise had been faithfully discharged. I recall that I felt, very strongly, that I had missed something in my secure "reserved occupation".

We unloaded next morning, about dawn, at a specially constructed "station" in the woods near the sector hospital. Our engine left us to go some substantial distance to find a turntable and my friend and I took one of many dawn walks in the Surrey woods. The dawn chorus was in full throat and the trees slender and grey with silvery leaves; but overhead the cloudless sky was darkened by aircraft as, the RAF having returned from its night raid on Germany, the US Air Force was assembling for its daylight assault. Layer upon layer of Flying Fortresses reached up into the pale blue of the sky, beautiful but sombre, to our eyes, knowing the losses suffered in these daylight raids. Nevertheless, there was a feeling of elation that morning – a certainty that the war was, at last, going our way and that VE Day could not be indefinitely postponed. In fact, the interval was to be much longer than we imagined and the setbacks and loss of life greater than seemed possible in the heady atmosphere of D Day + 1. But the foundation for VE Day had been laid, and it is still D Day which I recall most vividly.

Italian scenes

JAN BROD

The spring of 1945 in southern Italy was glorious. What a difference from the previous year, when the whole countryside was under a heavy layer of grey ashes from the recent eruption of Vesuvius, covering the trees, leaves, blossoms, and fields, and making the roads and footpaths in places impassable. At that time the war was still only at the other side of Naples and Capua, the battle of Cassino still raging. Now everything was different. The ashes were at least partly removed or gone, trees were in full bloom, and the war was pushed far away – to the other side of the Appenines, to the valley of the Po – and the hope of the final victory filled our hearts.

Seeing the sights

During the second week in April I got my regular leave and went to pass part of it in Rome where I intended to spend only three days, but the fascination of the Eternal City was such that I stayed on yet another day until the late afternoon of 12 April. I easily hitch hiked to Terni but dusk started to approach and most drivers were now reluctant to take unknown travellers. Finally, in clouds of dust, a jeep approached at top speed and almost passed me. Suddenly the driver – a British major – noticed my lifted thumb. He stopped abruptly, urged me to jump in "quickly, quickly", as he was expected before night fall in Ancona, some 140 miles away across the wild range of mountains. I was hardly seated before we moved at some 70–80 miles an hour on a twisting narrow road with steep rocks on one side and ravines and wild mountain streams on the other, bypassing Spoleto on top of a high hill. When, 45 minutes later, the major stopped to let me out in Foligno, he asked whether I was not scared of his wild driving through the numerous hairpins, assuring me that it was nothing as he was a racing driver in peacetime. The remaining nine miles in a taxi took me through unforgettably beautiful scenery with Assisi in the magic light of the last rays of the sun. During dinner in the officers' mess at the Subassio Hotel we were staggered by the unexpected radio news of the death of President Roosevelt.

I spent the whole of the next day sightseeing and remember even now, 40 years later, the unreal atmosphere on the top of the rocca (castle); had somebody told me that an angel had just descended next to me I would have believed him. Perugia, a walk beside Lake Trasimeno, and a short visit to Orvieto with the fantastic Lucca Signorelli frescoes in the cathedral ended my leave, and I returned next day to 103 General Hospital in Nocera Inferiore, in a picturesque mountain valley between Pompeii and Salerno.

Events now took a precipitate course. Every day a new victory and the fall of one or more places in the Po Valley and in Germany were announced. On 2 May the Germans capitulated in Italy; on 4 May the radio announced the surrender of the enemy armies in Germany to Montgomery. On Saturday 5 May, to celebrate the end of the war, I gave one of the regular gramophone record concerts in our hospital with English and Czech music (Elgar, Smetana, Dvořák) on the programme. Somehow, however, it seemed to be utterly unreal that the six years of dangers, anxieties, doubts, depression, and losses were over, and I had to be alone with the borrowed gramophone to think it over for myself to the sound, for the lack of anything more appropriate, of Brahms's second piano concerto, which one of my colleagues, Captain Roger (who unfortunately died very prematurely) carried around through his various stations in the theatre of war.

Next afternoon during ward rounds with the unforgettable Paul Wood (who for the past two years had been the OC of our medical division) the rumour reached us of the unconditional surrender of the Germans, which was confirmed the same evening by the radio. Disquieting news for me came only from Prague where the Germans were resisting and where street fighting broke out; but there also all was over within two days. On 8 May the whole staff of the hospital, together with the patients, celebrated VE Day by a thanksgiving mass under the open sky and by a dance with the nurses. On 13 May many of us went to nearby Salerno to see at the local theatre Verdi's *Masked Ball* with Benjamino Gigli as Ricardo

– unfortunately too fat at that late period of his life and with only short spells reminiscent of his fabulous voice.

Mistakes and misunderstandings

On the way back in the lorry I noticed that my right middle finger was sore. This increased next day and I started running a slight temperature. After showing my finger to Hedley Atkins (our surgical OC) and to Wood, I found myself admitted the same evening to the officers' ward. Next morning Wood examined me very carefully from top to toe, scrutinising my fingers and toes, my heart, and even my occular fundi, until I asked him whether he suspected an embolism from bacterial endocarditis. He gave a short laugh and said he was surprised I did not suspect it myself. Whereupon my blood was duly drawn for bacteriological culture and a thrice hourly very painful course of penicillin intramuscularly was started. At night I had hardly fallen asleep when I felt the sister drawing my mosquito net from underneath the mattress to give me a sting in my behind. Two days later the corporal from the laboratory, passing my bed, asked me how I was and when I said he probably knew better, he replied cheerfully, "Oh, the major said it's growing". The shock this gave me can be easily imagined. To live through the dangers of the war, the bombing of London, the torpedoing and sinking of our ship (the *Windsor Castle*), the front line, and then to perish miserably, when all was over by such a banal (in those days) illness! I said so to Wood later in the morning. His face flushed with anger and he wanted to know the source of my information. When I refused to give it, he went away, came back a couple of hours later, stretched out on the empty bed next to mine, and started to discuss various postwar topics, the teaching of medicine, research projects etc. This diverted my mind for a while from what I thought was my evil fate. Later the same day, Tony Hill (a boy with an ingenuous mind, a physiologist, a pupil of Samson Wright, whose company I liked very much) rushed to my bed, his face reddened and distorted with rage, called me a liar, and ran away without any explanation. I was dumbfounded. In the evening Maxwell Gardiner, a charming young Scottish member of our medical division, whom I often protected against Wood's unjustified attacks, explained to me what had happened. Wood blamed the major in charge of the laboratory for the indiscretion and the major's suspicion fell at once on Tony, who worked in the laboratory and whose friendship with me was known. He, therefore, had an awful row with him and Hill acted accordingly. No explanations to Gardiner or Wood helped as I did not want to let the corporal down.

I was transferred from the hospital a fortnight later to perhaps the loveliest place in the world, the Hotel Palumbo in Ravello (Richard Wagner, who spent his last summer holidays there before his death in 1882, wrote in the hotel guest book: "Klingsor's magic garden found"). When I came back, fully restored and confident at last that everything was a false alarm, Hill and Gardiner were gone so that I was unable to explain their error to them. I saw Hill over the heads of many people at a lecture by Professor Goormaghtigh in the Middlesex Hospital on 30 October 1946, but before I could push my way through to him after the lecture he was gone and I never succeeded in tracing his address. I also tried to contact Gardiner on one of my visits to Edinburgh but there was no answer to my call. Perhaps, if by any chance they read these lines, they will believe that I was never disloyal to our friendship.

Against regulations

The pressure of the routine work had now decreased and I began analysing the data of our study on acute glomerulonephritis which I had started with Wood's consent in spring 1944. As our routine laboratory was overtaxed I had to do the renal function tests, in the first place the weekly quantitative urine analyses, endogenous creatinine clearances, and, at longer intervals, the dilution and concentration tests, myself. The orderlies helped me to establish a small laboratory in the corner of my office: two improvised tables on trestles, a shelf for the reagents and distilled water from an irrigator, a sink made from a biscuit tin with a hole in the bottom draining into a bucket, and an old photoelectric colorimeter borrowed from Professor Califano at the Naples University department of chemistry. Wood also arranged that I could always take in a soldier with some minor ailment requiring daily therapy, like a backache, who could be trained to carry out the laboratory work under my guidance. And so originated one of the first studies on acute glomerulonephritis carried out with modern techniques on 66 patients, some of whom were followed up for six months, which was later published in the *American Journal of Medicine*.

One evening in June, as I was reading at the open window of my room, the commanding officer, Colonel Smith, stopped during his evening walk at my window for a chat. Suddenly he spotted some irregular equipment in the corner of my room and asked what it was. My heart stood still. What I was doing and what Wood had authorised was entirely against all regulations; the chronically ill patients, instead of being notified as "unfit to travel", should have been evacuated weeks or months ago to the UK. I stammered some explanation and the CO decided to come in and find out more. He sat in front of me listening and looking at my protocols. Then he left without a word and I rushed out to tell Wood that we both would probably be court martialled. Weeks passed, however, and nothing happened; then, at his farewell dinner, Colonel Smith gave a short speech and said he had put my name up for mention in despatches for research carried out under adverse conditions in the theatre of war. A few months later it came through.

It was at about the same time that Hedley Atkins's predecessor Lieutenant Colonel Bentley – later professor of plastic surgery at Newcastle upon Tyne – visited us on his way from Yugoslavia where he was temporarily attached to Tito's medical services to instruct them in the use of penicillin (having been the first successfully to treat open femur fractures with a primary suture and the antibiotic). After dinner he came to talk to me, told me some harrowing stories about life in Belgrade, about his arrest and near execution by the Yugoslav police and warned me of life in the eastern countries. I listened to him sceptically; anyway my home – Czechoslovakia – was in the very centre and not in the east of Europe. When, on my last leave in Italy at Lake Como, I was visited by my past CO from 220 Field Ambulance at the Garigliano front Colonel L F W Salmon – later senior ENT consultant at Guy's, who became a life long close friend, and who at that time was ADMS with the army HQ in Milan – he seemed very worried about postwar developments. During a trip on a rowing boat on the lake he expressed to me confidentially his fears that should I return to Czechoslovakia we might soon find ourselves on opposite sides of the fence. How right he was became clear to me only a few months later, when back in Prague. But that is a different story.

Strictly personal

R D CATTERALL

My personal VE Day was on 14 April 1945 when American tanks from General Patton's Third US Army advanced rapidly into central Germany along the autobahn from Weimar to Chemnitz. Some of them had been informed that there was a prisoner of war hospital at the Bethlehem Stift at Hohenstein-Ernstthal, a little village just south of the autobahn. A small force of one tank and two jeeps was despatched to investigate.

Unfortunately it ran into a group of German SS troopers and there was a sharp exchange of machine gun fire. A German was seriously wounded and two Australian medical orderlies from our hospital volunteered to take out our antiquated ambulance and bring him in. They were caught in the crossfire between the two groups and the ambulance was hit several times. Titch Foster, a corporal captured in Tobruk in 1941, was killed instantly and his companion was badly wounded in the leg. A few minutes later the main American force swept up the autobahn and there was no further fighting.

Later that morning, at 08.50 to be exact, a small group of us was standing by the main gate, which was unguarded for the first time. Two American tanks drove up and in the first was a battle stained Texan who fixed me with compassionate eyes and said, "Say boy, how long you been a prisoner?" "Four years," I replied hesitantly. "Gee," he said, "and you still alive." "I think so," I ventured, at which he disappeared into the inside of his tank and re-emerged holding a full bottle of Johnnie Walker whisky, which he placed firmly into my hands.

It was obvious that the dose would be homeopathic for the large numbers now gathering round the tank, so I gave it to the Scottish padre to distribute. He solved the problem by taking a huge swig himself and then passing the bottle round, saying repeatedly, "Don't forget the others". The bottle passed his way more than once before it was finally emptied.

My war started in 1939 when I volunteered to go to Finland to drive an ambulance in the winter war against the Russians. It included some action in Norway, internment in Sweden for six months, a long and complicated journey from Stockholm to Cairo by way of Moscow and Istanbul, and a few sorties in the western desert, before being sent to Greece early in 1941. Unfortunately the last destroyer, intended to evacuate us, did not come into the little port of Kalamata on the night of Tuesday 29 April 1941. The following morning units of the Wehrmacht occupied the town.

Dangerous moments

There are two major danger periods for prisoners of war, namely, the moment of capture and the moment of liberation. I was captured in the main street of Kalamata by a German lieutenant and two corporals in an armoured car. One of the corporals came over to me as I got out of the ambulance and pressed a light machine gun into my abdomen. He looked very young, even to me, and I could feel that his hand was trembling. So was mine. I was the first "enemy" he had encountered face to face. I mobilised a few words of schoolboy German and, once he had confirmed that I was not armed, he lowered the gun and we exchanged a mutual smile.

By February 1945 we could hear the guns of the Russian armies approaching the German frontiers, and our hospital, situated northeast of Dresden at Elsterhorst in Brandenberg, was in danger of being overrun. Heavy artillery fire could be heard at night and there was increasing aerial activity, reaching its height on 13 and 14 February with the sensational bombing of Dresden by the RAF and the US Air Force. We were awoken by the light of fires burning in the city nearly 40 miles away.

Suddenly, as the noise of the guns got even nearer, it was announced that all British prisoners were to be evacuated to the west, leaving the French, Poles, and other nationals behind. We were marched down to the railway and loaded into cattle trucks with equipment, food parcels, blankets, clothing, and all the other paraphernalia of a hospital. Although we were told our journey would last only one day our destination was not revealed. However, as a result of Allied bombing and strafing it took us six days to reach our initial destination, Hohenstein-Ernstthal, about 80 miles away. During all this time we were under constant threat from our own planes. It was bitterly cold, the ground was covered with snow, and food was short. Had it not been for Red Cross parcels the situation would have been serious. Fortunately, the more gravely ill of our patients had recently been repatriated through Lake Constance.

When we finally arrived at Hohenstein-Ernstthal we found it was mainly occupied by French doctors, orderlies, and patients. The majority were still quite uncertain as to where their loyalties lay and were basically Pétainist with only a few wholehearted supporters of de Gaulle. There were also some Americans captured in von Rundstedt's counter attack in the Ardennes, later known as the Battle of the Bulge. Their morale was very low and they segregated themselves from the others. We insisted that they ate communally with us, sharing all our food instead of each one hoarding little scraps with jealousy, resentment, and loneliness. By the time we were freed relationships and morale were good and many lasting friendships had been made.

Shortly before liberation the sadism of the Nazi regime was brought to our attention by the sight of a party of women Jews guarded by German women with whips. They marched past our hospital escorted by German soldiers with rifles and fixed bayonets. The Jewish women were struggling under heavy loads and had no proper footwear. They disappeared silently along the road to Chemnitz.

Welcome hospitality

The Americans evacuated all our patients to a US Army hospital in Ehrfurt and eventually home with remarkable speed. Within a few days we had no patients and no responsibilities and were destined to wait for air transport to fly us home. We were low on the list of priorities – it was over two weeks before we finally arrived back in the UK, one of us in the rear gunner's seat of a Lancaster bomber. Meanwhile, in the military barracks in Ehrfurt the Americans offered us lavish hospitality, which was most welcome after four years in "the bag".

When the real VE Day finally dawned and the Germans signed the unconditional surrender I was still waiting to go home. I was also experiencing the charms and joys of feminine company, of which I had been deprived for over four years. When I first met the nurses of the American field hospital situated near Weimar I felt clumsy and ill at ease. I rapidly fell in love with a dazzling lieutenant from Boston, who became the object of my dreams and the most beautiful girl in the world. She understood the difficulties of adjusting to normal living and gradually brought me back to a feeling of comfort and assurance in female company.

In the evening there was a huge turkey and cranberry sauce dinner and dance to which I was invited; but a form of agoraphobia took hold of me and I was reluctant to go to it. Instead, my lieutenant organised a quiet dinner for two, my first bottle of champagne for five years, and her undivided attention for me alone. My VE Day was very private, full of tenderness, and very therapeutic.

Taste of freedom

Nearly 40 years have elapsed since the Allied victory in the second world war in Europe. This is the lifetime of a generation, and almost half the present population was not even born. The war marks a watershed of national and personal experience, separating those who lived through it from those who did not.

Human memory for emotions, moods, and reactions is usually shortlived and it is difficult to recall nuances of feeling. No doubt immediately after release everyone felt overjoyed and greatly relieved. Nevertheless, one of our patients developed an acute paranoid reaction and saw Germans under his bed, in cupboards, and all around him. Despite very close nursing surveillance he successfully committed suicide shortly after liberation and five years after being captured.

Most of us were underweight, tired easily, had impaired concentration and a poor memory; we felt awkward on meeting strangers and had a strong desire to be alone; in some cases there was true agoraphobia with unwillingness to meet people at all. Opinions as to the value of having been a prisoner varied greatly. Some thought that captivity was a pure loss and it was a disgrace to have been captured at all. Others felt they had benefited, especially when educational and cultural facilities were available. There was also the value of close contact with prisoners of other nationalities, and opportunities to observe all types of men under duress.

As for me, some of the most striking memories of returning home were the joys of clean sheets, new clothes, tomato sandwiches and china tea on an English lawn, freedom of movement, and privacy. The experience of captivity was an endowment and changed the whole of my life and outlook. It even made me take up medicine.

Down under

CYRIL CLARKE

In October 1944 Féo (my wife) and I were on leave in the Lake District – a short distance from Liverpool where I had a job as medical specialist (roughly the equivalent of a senior registrar) in the Royal Naval Auxiliary Hospital, Seaforth. Previously, since the beginning of the war, I had been for three years in the hospital ship HMHS *Amarapoora*. She was stationed initially in Scapa but later, after the landings, she made trips to north Africa. Coming home from one of these I had to look after a number of US Army psychiatric patients. They terrified me but I solved the problem by recruiting a bodyguard of German prisoners of war (under a sergeant major called Adolf) and they ensured my safety.

To return to that October. After tramping the hills we got back to our lakeland digs and there was a telegram. I opened it in trepidation – "Proceed to Royal Naval Hospital, Sydney, Australia". Extrasystoles + +. I had endured (that is mostly enjoyed) four years of war, but although the situation in Europe was improving there seemed no chance that Japan would ever pack up, and I felt that I should end my days in the southern hemisphere. But my headmaster had told me, "The secret of a happy life is to live dangerously", so I did not argue – and it sounded a good job.

Advance to Australia

So in November 1944 we sailed away from Liverpool in the *Empress of Scotland* (J1) bound for Sydney westabout, via Panama. We were the advance party and were eight officers to a cabin. Reason: the top deck was occupied by the new governor of New South Wales, complete with wife, children, and nannies + +. Were we bolshie?

The *Empress* did 23 knots, and after a destroyer escort down St George's Channel away we went at full bat – too fast for the submarines. She was a great ship but, awkwardly, had been christened the *Empress of Japan*. For obvious reasons this had become unsuitable, but there had not been time to substitute the cabin notices, which all remained in Japanese. The Panama Canal was fantastic – efficient and quiet, quite different from the navvy shouting that went on at Suez. But the prickly heat was terrible – we just lay and gasped.

We made Sydney in 28 days and here it nearly all ended. None of us had seen the lights of a city for five years, and there was Sydney lit up for Christmas. The ship was going slightly astern preparatory to anchoring and there was a cross wind; everyone, of course, rushed to the landward side to get the view – at least 2000 of us. There came a frantic shout from the bridge as the *Empress* began to heel over – "Balance the ship" or its equivalent. We did, and she righted, but I had not realised that 23 000 tons could behave like a dinghy.

The hospital was not ready for us – it had only been recently evacuated by the Americans, who had gone up north – so we stayed in a famous family hotel, Petty's (now pulled down), where we must have spent about a month. At a reception party we had our first casualty: our toothie (I forget his name) slid down and off the bannisters and broke his neck, but happily survived.

Hospitality + + from the Prince Alfred Hospital (grand rounds every Sunday morning, led by Kempson Maddox), and an extraordinary party on arrival where, to my astonishment, everyone was talking French. Reason: Kempson was entertaining a party from Numea (French Caledonia).

The war seemed miles away, though the Sydneyites frequently reminded us how a Japanese submarine had shelled their harbour. Somehow the sub had got through the defences but, unlike Prien at Scapa, it did not get out again.

The hospital job was marvellous, all the main specialties represented and well staffed, and I learnt medicine at the rate of knots. Navy discipline was admirable and I had entire clinical freedom, except on one memorable occasion. I had under my care a most attractive VAD with a tuberculous pleural effusion. When she recovered I made the standard recommendation that she be invalided home, but I was told by a surgeon commander that she would do better if we kept her in the Antipodes. The reasoning was biased, but I was only a two striper so I had to cave in.

Ian Sneddon, the Sheffield dermatologist, came out in J2; we became great friends and bought a dinghy which we sailed in Botany Bay. The sailing both there and in Sydney Harbour was marvellous and we raced VJs, 16 footers, and watched the incredible Sydney Harbour 18s with 2000 feet of sail – but they were old fashioned and to windward would be seen off by a 14 foot International. Betting was not legal, but there was a bookies' launch which followed each race and the crew had numbers on their backs like footballers.

Nearly the end

VE Day came and passed us by. Eternity still seemed ahead, but about July 1945 Surgeon Captain Lambert Rogers, who was our neurosurgical specialist, told us we should be home by Christmas (he was obviously in the know) and in August came Hiroshima and Nagasaki and the war was over – just as we had got organised.

VJ Day I shall never forget. There was a strong breeze and Ian and I were celebrating by a sail in Botany Bay. A gust, and over we went. I knew it – after six years of war we should be "taken" by a shark at the moment of victory. But the shadow of the sail is apparently protective and we managed to swim ashore, dragging the boat with us.

There was more to come: a medical spin off. The Hong Kong beri-beri patients (poor things) came to us and we saw the most fantastic array of CNS problems. Ian and I wrote a paper about their nutritional neuropathies and had a film made of the clinical features. Another spin off was the butterflies. There were monarchs and swallowtails everywhere and my love for them returned – but that is a story on its own.

I came home in a P & O troopship and we had a moving experience in Fremantle, for there we landed hundreds of Aussie servicemen who were coming home from fighting the war up north. The town band was there to meet us, and back it came at 5 am the next morning when we sailed for Southampton – and there were cheering crowds as well to see us off. The Japs had been beaten and the millennium was ahead.

Twenty three years later I flew into Perth and as I landed there was still cheering. I thought, "It can't be for me". It wasn't. It was for the Crown Prince and Princess of Japan. O tempora, O mores.

Homecoming

Arriving in Southampton at Christmas time, in pouring rain, the brave boys came home to no band and to a perishing winter. I made my way home to Leicester and joined my family (Charles Clarke, aged 2, said "kangaloo" to me) and we all stayed with my mother – me a brave boy with pockets full of glowing flimsies and a story of marvellous jobs, plus our POW film. Everyone would be wanting me. But slowly it dawned that there were many others with equal credentials, and for three months I was jobless and my mother's gas bill was £20 – Féo and I used to sit for hours in front of the spare room fire scouring the *BMJ* and *Lancet*. There was nothing doing at Guy's – the dean suggested general practice at Emsworth (the sailing there was excellent) – and I was turned down at Guildford. But in March 1946 there was a registrar's job going at the Queen Elizabeth Hospital at Birmingham. I applied, got my old chiefs John Ryle and C P Symonds to back me, and landed it after a tussle. But was I medically qualified? Could I *prove* it? I was baffled, but it turned out that my predecessor (the best registrar they had ever had) was a physiotherapist.

I loved the QE. The salary was £300 a year and Féo and I and the three children lived in digs in a working class area and I bicycled each day to the hospital and never took a day off.

The horizon got brighter. I had had my sights on Liverpool because of my year's service there, and about July was interviewed by Henry Cohen. I landed a consultant job at the Northern Hospital and started work on 1 September 1946.

The next 37 years are in the red book.

Painting the town

JOHN CLUBB

The eminent urologist Mr Yates-Bell and his minion registrars and housemen sprayed us liberally with what we hoped, in retrospect, was nothing more sinister than soda water. This urological baptism heralded the start of VE Day and somewhat dampened our plans to take the "mickey" out of the consultant staff. They had got the blow in first.

We had been sitting in the refectory at Leatherhead Hospital, drinking what in wartime passed for coffee, and feeling that an era had come to an end; rejoicing that the war in Europe was over, and wondering what life would be like in peacetime. Because so many doctors were in the armed services, the senior medical students at King's had been given responsibilities and opportunities normally available only to newly qualified doctors. King's students were split among Denmark Hill in London, Horton Hospital in Epsom, and Leatherhead Hospital. Far from suffering from this disruption, our clinical education was widened by having to deal with the casualties of war from the services and civilian life.

Descent on London

Abandoning plans to do anything collectively outrageous, we changed into dry clothes and went our separate ways. I decided to walk to Epsom and catch a train to Wimbledon, where my fiancee Elizabeth, also a medical student, lived. All the pubs on the way to Epsom were thronged with happy, singing people, and my recollection is that pubs stayed open all day and night. Elizabeth's family had a definite army background. Her father had served in the Boer war and in both world wars, and he was now the head of the explosives department at the Home Office. Her brother David was a regular officer in the Royal Artillery, a youthful veteran of Dunkirk and north Africa, recently returned from a German POW camp. When I arrived many of their friends were there, including an attractive Wren, Jill, and Stephen, who was a paratrooper. Stephen was planning a VE night descent on London, not by parachute but by train. I found myself being indoctrinated in the art of jumping out of a moving train by numbers, as though from an aircraft, and landing in one piece on the platform. When he judged us all to be reasonably proficient we set out armed with smoke canisters, thunderflashes, and, above all, Stephen's tremendous personality.

There were eight of us in the group and we spent the time in the train between Wimbledon and Waterloo in further rehearsal for the drop. He had us all lined up in a row holding on to the luggage rack, whilst he lay full length on the rack supervising the descent. As we approached Waterloo the train slackened speed and we were made to leap out in order. Number one in pride of place was Elizabeth, who landed on the platform, to my relief, without breaking her neck or anything else. I had barely time to take that in before I was shoved out, followed by the army, navy, marines, and civilians remaining in the carriage. We all picked ourselves up in time to see Stephen descend sedately from the compartment, letting off two thunderflashes as he did so. This caused a certain amount of consternation in the station and we left hurriedly in the direction of Waterloo Bridge, making our way along the Strand in the direction of Trafalgar Square.

Joy and laughter

The crowd grew thicker. "Keep behind me and form a chain," said Stephen, lighting a smoke canister, and he charged through the throng, which opened before him like the Red Sea in front of Moses. We came to one of the lions around Nelson's column opposite the National Gallery. Stephen climbed on to the back of the lion and began to auction off the gallery and all its paintings. "Who will make me an offer?" he said. Elizabeth's younger brother Martin, a schoolboy, bid half a crown. The bidding progressed in leaps and bounds before the gallery and contents were sold to an American master sergeant for 100 dollars. He was told to take the money to the director of the gallery next morning to collect his purchase.

Leaping down from the lion, Stephen led us to a boarded up statue near St Martin-in-the-Fields with the object of continuing the auction of the sights of London. By this time, however, we had attracted the attention of the police and they had formed a cordon around us. Unconcerned at the presence of the law, Stephen shouted, "What am I bid for this pride of policemen – all in excellent condition?" The crowd loved this, and bids came fast and furious. In no time at all they were knocked down, in a manner of speaking, to the selfsame master sergeant for another 100 bucks. Before he could collect his purchases the "pride" sheepishly shuffled off, deciding that we were mad rather than drunk. Since Stephen was in fact a teetotaller their diagnosis was correct.

The victorious auctioneer had by this time acquired a vast crowd and, with our help, scaled one of the recruiting hoardings in the square. There, bathed in the light of mobile searchlights brought into London, Stephen began an oration. "Tonight we are celebrating a famous victory. A victory won by one army alone, and to that army we owe our lives and liberty." The American master sergeant didn't much like the sound of this and neither did 50 other GIs with him. They started to climb up the hoarding with murderous intent. "For goodness sake tell Stephen to shut up," whispered Elizabeth to me. But it was too late. "Which army won the war?" yelled Stephen. "I'll tell you which. It wasn't the American army. It wasn't the French army. It wasn't the Poles." The master sergeant had nearly reached the top of the hoarding by this time and the tension in the crowd was rising. "The army which won this war," cried Stephen, pointing to the recruiting poster below him, "the army which won this war was the Women's Land Army." The relief of tension was instantaneous and the crowd roared with laughter at the joke as the Americans climbed down from the lynching party and joined in the applause.

. . . When the lights go up

Piccadilly Circus was the next stop, where our smoke canisters disrupted a group on top of one of the air raid shelters. They were celebrating VE night in their own inimitable, not to say intimate, style. A girl stood up, naked except for a cigarette holder. As if by design or even magic a roving searchlight focused on target, joined swiftly by yet another searchlight. The crowd gazed astonished at a sight more usually seen at the nearby Windmill Theatre. Even more action packed, for in those days stage nudes were static. This shapely nude was neither static nor sober, and began to pirouette around, swaying and waving her cigarette holder to all and sundry. She had been entertaining about half a dozen of our gallant allies, who cascaded off the roof of the air raid shelter in various stages of undress, leaving her as the star attraction, until the searchlights moved on. We also moved away, as a rumour spread through the crowd that the Royal Family and Winston Churchill were due to appear on the balcony at Buckingham Palace.

Our invaluable smoke enabled us to get right up to the gates of the palace, where we had a superb view of the King and Queen, the two princesses, and Winston Churchill and his wife, Clemmie. We sang all the usual patriotic songs and cheered ourselves hoarse. After numerous appearances the King and Queen waved their final farewells and the crowds began to disperse happily for home. We were feeling tired by this time and walked back down the Mall, climbed the Duke of York's steps and found ourselves outside the Athenaeum Club. "They might put us all up for the night here," said Stephen.

We did not think that the Athenaeum was a very likely resting place, especially as there were three ladies among us. Nothing daunted, Stephen rang the doorbell. A venerable retainer eventually appeared, listened to our request for lodging with great courtesy, and politely but firmly stated that we could not enter as we were not members. After he had locked and bolted the imposing doors we decided to extend the embargo placed on us to the general public. Removing the barriers and notice boards from a nearby road works, we carried them back to the Athenaeum and barricaded it off with "No entry" signs.

By this time we really were tired and walked back to Waterloo, where we slept on the wooden benches until a milk train at 5 am took us back to Wimbledon, weary but feeling that it had all been worth while and memorable.

At any cost

K W DONALD

VE Day was no surprise; we had known for some time that Germany and its armed forces were no longer able to hold the thrusts of the Allied armies from all directions. Nevertheless, the reality of Germany's surrender was still a wonderful lightening of the spirit after so many years. The impossible had come to pass. The brutal and perverted Nazi regime, supported by the most formidable fighting machine yet known in the world, was destroyed, probably for ever. The real possibility, and to some the certainty, of the whole human race being overwhelmed by this monstrous and barbaric regime had disappeared. Japan remained a distant but powerful enemy who would inevitably be defeated but at great cost in human lives. Winston Churchill, like a stern headmaster, had agreed that there was some justification for a brief celebration but there must be no relaxation, no rest until Japan too was conquered. We would have to screw our courage to the sticking point once more.

As we duly celebrated and toasted victory (it was my wife's birthday as well) I looked back over the past six years. War, with its dangers, tensions, and austerity had become a way of life.

The most outstanding memory was of our attitude in 1940 and 1941, when a whole nation ignored the obvious and refused to think in terms of surrender; possible defeat, yes, but never surrender. There were no further discussions about the situation, not even with oneself. The exhilaration of intense danger and of total commitment was indeed a heady wine.

Lost harvest

In every war each person had unique memories which remain fresh and undulled by the passage of time: the noise of the passing of a

16 in shell from the *Scharnhorst*, like an oldfashioned tram roaring down a high terraced road; again, the 5 in shell penetrating the ship's side and the hull sounding as if it was made of rubber; the explosion of an ammunition ship which was so appallingly violent that one hardly heard it.

War gives one strange opportunities. When I was a surgeon lieutenant in Norway I agreed to buy the whole of the cod liver oil harvest of northern Norway, which was stored in great tanks in Svolvaer, Lofoten Islands. I forget how much there was and how many millions I agreed to pay on behalf of the British government. I sent an urgent message to Skjelfiord where the senior naval officer's ship was lying. Incredibly, it was passed through the appropriate channels to the highest level and it was apparently agreed that a clean tanker should be sent to collect it. The file stuck on somebody's desk and when all was ready the British had just left Norway. It was a sad loss. I never received any condemnation (or praise) for my presumption (or initiative).

When the Germans had retaken Narvik we had to run the gauntlet with the wounded of the first destroyer battle of Narvik from Gravdal, Vestvågöy, to Harstad in a Norwegian fishing boat. We were wearing rollneck sweaters and miscellaneous trousers, a deliberately ambiguous naval uniform. It finally happened half way there: we passed, about a quarter of a mile away, a boat laden with German infantry sitting in regular rigid rows, proceeding in the opposite direction. We waved to them enthusiastically and they waved back, delighted and, perhaps, surprised to meet such a friendly reception. They did not stop. If they had done so it would have been an even longer war for some.

Another vivid memory was of the last really ideal night (according to Admiralty) for the German invasion across the English Channel. The tides, the moon, and weather were all perfect. Our destroyer moved slowly and quietly through the calm dark waters. The engines stopped. There was only the gentle lapping of water. We listened, we waited, we listened. They never came. They were preparing for their attack in the east, where a dreadful nemesis awaited them.

War under water

Later I joined an even stranger war of submarines and many other underwater activities. With the stimulus of war the heavy helmeted and booted diver of the past was liberated into a whole variety of free swimming divers, unattached by air pipes or lifelines, carrying their own gas and often wearing flippers. The emergence of the charioteers (riding torpedoes), frogmen, mine disposal divers, and baby submarines (X craft) with divers who could leave and return to the craft, was a fascinating period of research, development, and training. The Italians had opened the score with a dashing human torpedo attack on Alexandria harbour where they gravely damaged two battleships. The greatest success of our X craft was the crippling of the mighty ship the *Tirpitz* in Altenfjord in September 1943. The price paid was very high but the *Tirpitz* never became fully operational again.

There was, as always, no shortage of volunteers for these most dangerous and sometimes almost suicidal missions. They were a very mixed bag from all sorts of professions and backgrounds. There were as many introverts as extroverts and most had a high degree of intelligence. Appropriate breathing apparatus and gases had to be developed and tested for each particular task. Those attacking heavily guarded harbours or coastal defences had to breath oxygen so that no excess gas was vented and giveaway bubbles caused on the surface. Oxygen was found to be toxic under water at depths as shallow as 30 feet. Various mixtures of oxygen and nitrogen could be calculated for use at different depths and with varying degrees of activity.

I was incredibly fortunate to have a highly intense and unorthodox training in hyperbaric medicine from J B S Haldane for a few months. A regular team of "experimental" divers was required, again all volunteers. These men were under pressure in tanks, chambers, docks, and even in the open sea five days a week for over two years. Fortunately none was killed or permanently damaged in any way. The human torpedoes had some tragic losses and some successes but it became more and more difficult for these men to penetrate harbour defences and attach their explosive warhead to the keel or hull of enemy ships.

The British frogmen were the first operational frogmen in the world. They used oxygen but did not dive to any significant depth except for very short periods. They were employed in a quite remarkable variety of commando type operations. Some were carried by baby submarines and emerged near enemy coasts to survey shore and beach defences as well as collecting mud and sand samples and assessing the weight bearing properties of the beach.

These were very individual warriors in their dangerous missions to attack harbours, dock gates, bridges, floating docks, and warships. After they had left their mother submarine or ship all one could do was wait and, perhaps, pray for their safe return.

One interesting clinical point emerged when developing the frogmen. A number became confused or even unconscious when swimming, and some were lost. We finally discovered that their oxygen uptake could be at levels equivalent to those of cross country skiing (4–5 l/min) and that these men were overloading their carbon dioxide absorbent canisters. Carbon dioxide in the inspired gas increased dramatically and they were anaesthetising themselves with their own body gases. This was part of the background that led up to my proposition in the *Lancet* in 1949 that patients in obstructive respiratory failure could suffer carbon dioxide narcosis when breathing oxygen – an idea that was, at first, violently opposed.

Irresistible danger

Mine disposal and the collection, dismantling, and analysis of new types of mine was another hazardous underwater activity. This naval branch was always leavened by a considerable number of Australians, who appeared to find its terrible danger completely irresistible. A considerable number of these mining experts had to be trained to organise and supervise large diving operations. I still remember teaching diving techniques and physiology on a hot summer's day to an attentive row of George Crosses and George Medals. How men who lived in such constant peril could concentrate on such matters as blood gases, hypoxia, the gas laws, the mechanism of reducing and demand valves, etc, etc, baffled me. On reflection, however, if the proximity of death concentrates the mind, these amazing men's minds were surely much concentrated.

The famous P parties of individual soft helmeted counterlung divers, who breathed appropriate proportions of oxygen and nitrogen for work at different depths, were greatly in evidence on and after D Day. They were able to travel rapidly to, say, a harbour in groups of up to 30. In a few minutes they would be searching the bottom of a basin, working on a grid, for timed charges which the enemy left as unwelcome souvenirs. Every inch had to be covered but they could find a silver coin if the bottom was not too muddy. It was a great day when the US forces sent for British P parties to "sanitise" newly captured Cherbourg before the ships came in. Our delight was because we had such a high regard for American underwater work and it was nice to be ahead just on this occasion.

*   *   *

These were some of my memories on VE Day. At this present time many people appear to doubt that all the courage, ingenuity, sacrifice, and suffering were really worth while and think that Europe was merely continuing its centuries old habit of self destruction. Yet those of us who have lived and grown old are still totally certain that almost the whole world had to be saved, at any cost, from a most dreadful tyranny.

The end of the beginning

J A DUDGEON

My recollections of VE Day are vivid indeed, for two reasons. First, because it was the day that I was married; and, second, because it was the day that my leave was cancelled. When I had joined the Territorial Army in 1936 I had been issued with a small booklet entitled *Advice to Young Officers*. The first piece of advice read, "Ask for leave at all times and in all places, and in the end you acquire a right to it". My previous good luck clearly did not prevail in May 1945, and, as I shall suggest later, I consider that the then Prime Minister was in part responsible.

Everyone in London, and indeed throughout the country, was in jubilant mood. Driving through London on that lovely May evening was an experience never to be forgotten. It was also hazardous. I recollect trying to navigate the car down St James's Street (you could drive down in those days). We had by that time acquired two Wrens perched on the roof, and two sailors on the bonnet, and having not so long before been navigation officer to my battalion in the western desert I had at least learned the need for a clear view ahead. The presence of the navy aboard made this difficult, but the Wrens were very sweet.

Uneasy mood

As far as I was concerned VE Day marked the end of the beginning. It had all begun 11 years earlier at Trinity College, Cambridge, where I had first met Elston Grey-Turner. We became great personal friends and our friendship was to last for 50 years, spanning medicine, life in the TA, the City, and the Society of Apothecaries, until his untimely death early this year. Little did we know throughout those idyllic and magical days at Trinity

59

(1934–8) that evil men were among us in Cambridge – Blunt, Burgess, Maclean, Philby and the like; but, as Trevor-Roper (now Lord Dacre) has described in his article "The acts of the Apostles", this was the plan.* After the furore of the Oxford Union debate of February 1933 Oxford may have appeared a rather sensitive area for subversive activities to Stalin, so what better and more unlikely location for such traitorous work than Trinity.

I had never heard of the "Apostles", and indeed I wonder if many of my contemporaries had; certainly Elston had not until we discussed Lord Dacre's article only a year ago. On the other hand, we were well aware of the open support for the Spanish civil war from men such as John Cornford, who was to die in that war, and others. The mood of the country at the time was uneasy and the unrealistic protagonists of pacifism received much attention. The government, under Stanley Baldwin, took it seriously, as the Incitement to Disaffection Bill was introduced into parliament in 1934 to protect service personnel from subversive activities. It was a direct result of frequent interruptions by agitators to sign petitions against this bill that I took a train to London and joined the London Rifle Brigade, and was subsequently one of the first officers commissioned by King Edward VIII in January 1936.

Real and imaginary difficulties

So much for the prologue, and now for VE Day and the events immediately surrounding it. At the second Quebec conference in September 1944, Roosevelt and Churchill had agreed to operation "Dracula", the code name for the seaborne invasion of southern Burma proposed by Mountbatten, supreme commander SEAC. In order to ease the strain on the Fourteenth Army driving south towards Mandalay with its lines of communication greatly overextended, a northward thrust from Rangoon was essential. This could only come from the sea across the Bay of Bengal. At the time medical casualties were heavy – Churchill had expressed alarm at the extent, 248 000 in Burma in the first six months of 1944. Malaria and scrub typhus were important causes of disease; with the former some form of prophylaxis in the form of mepacrine was available, but little could be done to afford protection against mite borne scrub typhus other than the use of insecticides. In 1943–4 it was clear that scrub typhus was one of the most serious medical

*New York Review of Books, 31 March 1983.

60

problems after malaria. A total of 5000 cases had occurred in the Fourteenth Army in Burma in 1944, with 350 deaths, and in 1944 the case mortality was 19.5% in some units. The advance of the Fourteenth Army southwards and the northerly thrust proposed in "Dracula" would take place through heavily infected scrub typhus areas. What could be done?

By early 1944, Forrest Fulton, then at the MRC laboratories at Hampstead, had shown that mice previously inoculated with a formalised inactivated suspension of cotton rat lungs infected with *Rickettsiae tsutsugamushi*, could be protected against challenge inoculation with the virulent rickettsiae. On the basis of this slender evidence a few doses of the "scrub typhus vaccine" were despatched to Dr R Lewthwaite, director of scrub typhus research in SEAC. This was in the autumn of 1944 and was intended for a "clinical trial". As far as I know this never took place, but what did happen was that in November 1944 a signal from HQ SEAC reached the War Office "requesting" 100 000 doses of scrub typhus vaccine as a top priority by August 1945. It may have been coincidence that at the time Churchill had written various memoranda about methods of defeating the Japanese, and in one he wrote, "All the alternatives should be examined in a hopeful spirit, resolute to overcome the real difficulties and brush away the still more numerous imaginary difficulties which always weigh in action".

The problems of producing a vaccine against scrub typhus were immense, apart from the fact that there was little evidence that it would work. There were no production facilities or trained staff such as now exist at the MRE Porton Down, and the stark fact was that *R tsutsugamushi* was one of the most lethal pathogens as far as laboratory workers were concerned.

Operation "Tyburn"

Such simple matters were there to be overcome, and as far as the PM was concerned the production of scrub typhus vaccine and the construction of the Mulberry harbours were of paramount importance. The Wellcome Foundation undertook to produce the vaccine for the Ministry of Supply, for the use of the army, under the aegis of the Medical Research Council. Such a complicated administrative arrangement would now appear to have all the ingredients of an assignment to catastrophe. The late Major General Poole and

61

Lieutenant Colonel Benstead at the War Office made all the necessary administrative arrangements. The operation was assigned a code name, special operation "Tyburn", as a top secret operation, which certainly had the effect of overcoming any difficulties as they arose. A site was chosen for the vaccine production unit at Frant, near Tunbridge Wells in Kent. Two field companies of Royal Engineers started on the foundations on 14 January 1945, and the buildings were completed on 4 May 1945, three weeks ahead of schedule. Laboratory staff had to be recruited from the services and the ATS. Ninety volunteered; they received a fortnight's training in laboratory procedures, and were then put to work on handling this highly pathogenic organism. They did a fine job.

The vaccine – if it could merit such a term – was produced from the lungs of cotton rats inoculated intranasally under anaesthesia. When they succumbed in a few days' time to pneumonia their lungs were removed, emulsified, and clarified by centrifugation, and this crude preparation constituted the vaccine. Formaldehyde was added in sufficient quantity to inactivate the rickettsia and a little extra for safety. After tests for potency and safety, which would be considered outrageously inadequate by any committee on the safety of medicines, the vaccine was ampouled and released.

The cotton rats had to be flown to England from America by Air Transport Command as at the time there was no breeding colony in the country. Elaborate precautions had to be taken to prevent contaminated air getting into the atmosphere. The risks were great, but the operation worked and only three laboratory infections occurred. These patients and one other all survived, two of them having received a massive inoculation. All four had been vaccinated, possibly the best proof that the vaccine had some effect, as clinical trials later on produced results of doubtful validity.

In October 1944 Churchill signalled Mountbatten that "Dracula" must be postponed until the autumn of 1945. By April 1945 the Fourteenth Army had reached the plains north of Mandalay and on 4 May Rangoon was reoccupied. On 7 May Montgomery accepted the surrender of the German army groups in the north and on 9 May Tedder, on behalf of Eisenhower, signed the final armistice with all German forces in Europe.

VE Day was on 8 May. Vaccine production started on 6 May and operation "Tyburn" was in full swing by 9 May, the day the campaign in Burma was over. Leave was cancelled to ensure a steady flow of vaccine. By September 1945, after the capitulation of Japan, 201.9 litres of vaccine had been produced and shipped to SEAC. A great deal was lost in transit to India, and we shall never know whether the fruits of our labours would have protected our troops. The strictly limited clinical trials were not altogether encouraging, but fortunately now scrub typhus responds well to chemotherapy. Nevertheless, it was a momentous undertaking, stirred on by decisions of those in high places, and well worth the effort.

Experience of a lifetime

DALE FALCONER

I must tell the truth: I had a wonderful war, for I was young and single and there was so much going on in these years. Each day provided its happiness, fear, or sadness. They were my salad days. And we did not think of ourselves all the time, as seems to be the characteristic of today, but rather of others who might be in need of support. All of us were nationalised into one great organisation with a single determination to overthrow the Nazi regime. We understood one another.

To be a surgeon lieutenant in the RNVR was advantageous. Often we felt sorry for the army, for we had warm cabins with running water (hot and cold) and a dry bunk. There was no mud or dust at sea and we were victualled regularly with hot food. Above all we enjoyed the somewhat risky privilege of sailing the world. It was the experience of a lifetime.

Medicine afloat

I remember sailing from Scapa Flow to welcome the first American naval task force which was coming across the Atlantic. The weather was so foul that at first we could not find the Americans. When we sighted them they reported the loss of an admiral overboard, and we had to escort the famous carrier USS *Wasp* straight to the Clyde for repair of her storm damage.

In the dread earlier days of the war I served in a cruiser with the Eastern Fleet. The Japanese navy had penetrated round the south of Ceylon, and although one day our opposing fleets were only 200 miles apart we never met. This was fortunate, for our C in C, Admiral Somerville, flew his flag in HMS *Warspite*, an old first world war battleship with a top speed of only 24 knots, and he was far too brave for my liking. On the Indian Ocean my surgical highlight was an appendicectomy. My boss the surgeon commander gave ether and chloroform by rag and bottle, and the entire convoy altered course into the wind for half an hour to steady the ship.

Forty years ago I received my first ever supply of penicillin to treat a young Wren who was dying of septicaemia. I gave it intravenously every two hours and her recovery was immediate. Some thirty ships' doctors from the base at Londonderry came to my sick quarters just to look at and smell the miraculous substance.

En route to South Africa we put in to Freetown for oil. No one went ashore, for we spent only six hours at the oil terminal, which was at the end of a pipeline and some 500 yards off the shore. At sea two days later one of the sailors developed a high temperature. At Cape Town they told me he had malaria. The diagnosis had not occurred to me, for it must take a very determined *Anopheles* to travel so far in one direction even along an oil pipe.

While in Johannesburg I had the opportunity of visiting Baragwanath Hospital, to which hundreds of our servicemen from the middle and far eastern forces had been invalided with pulmonary tuberculosis. It was a disturbing occasion for I realised that half these patients would not survive. Before leaving I was taken to the ward containing 11 of my fellow surgeon lieutenants. All had cavities which they showed to me on their *x* rays.

Great men and others

One night we received a signal with instructions to intercept a German hospital ship repatriating wounded from Salonika to Trieste and which was suspected of carrying senior officers who were fit and well. We stopped her off Crete and I was sent over in the motor boat to find out who was on board. The ship was crowded with very sick soldiers and everywhere there was a stench. Alone I was quite unable to determine who was who on board and we were ordered to Alexandria to land all passengers. I spent the night on the bridge talking with the master. He told me that his home in Hamburg had been destroyed by bombers and also that our British aircraft sank hospital ships. Eventually his hospital ship left Alexandria for Trieste albeit without any wounded on board. Two days later we heard that she had been sunk in the Adriatic by our air force stationed at Bari – a case of mistaken identity.

Only once did I encounter the great men of the war. We took Field Marshal Alexander, the commander in chief of the Allied armies in Italy, from Taranto to Athens because the weather forecast was so bad that they would not allow him to fly. Our tiny ship, a hunt class destroyer, was no flagship, and so the captain gave over his cabin to the field marshal, and the two generals who accompanied him were given my sick bay; one had the examination couch and the other the operating table. Overnight the sea became bumpy and they must have been uncomfortable, but next morning all three were determined to shave. A daily shave seemed to be a point of honour in the army. As we approached Piraeus, Alexander divulged that they were going to meet Churchill, who would be arriving by air. He had discounted the weather forecast, although later we could see the turbulence written all over Eden's face. To complete the party Macmillan, the minister resident in north west Africa, arrived magnificently in HMS *Ajax*. It was Christmas Day 1944 and there was great trouble in Athens. As we lay at anchor they started to fire mortar bombs at us, and we had to move further offshore.

During the closing months of the war in Europe we had been with convoys taking supplies from the Thames across to the Scheldt estuary and shielding them from enemy gunboats, which would appear from nowhere during the night. When finally the enemy had withdrawn we sailed up to Rotterdam, and to celebrate we gave a tea party for the Dutch children of a nearby school. They gobbled our bananas and chocolate, which they had never seen in their lives before. Their schoolmaster and his wife sat beside each other in the ward room and told me what the war in Holland had meant to them. They had no children of their own. As a condition of remaining with his wife he had agreed to be castrated.

Into the unknown

Such was the panorama of events in which one was caught. The war had been so compelling that I feared for the future, and when VE Day came I and my shipmates remained quietly on board off Southend pier. We did not go ashore to celebrate. At night we saw the lights over London playing and rejoicing in the sky, yet after years in the Royal Navy we could only wonder what would become of us.

On 7 March 1946 I was released from naval service. I put on my demob suit of clothes and my trilby hat and glanced in the mirror. After the smart navy blue I had to laugh. Now I was leaving my first salaried job for the unknown. There was no national health service in which to take refuge. From then on I was on my own.

*   *   *

Elston Grey-Turner was a young man who shone in time of war. Many years later there were those postwar colleagues who would smile at "the Colonel". As a part time territorial soldier he had attained the rank of full colonel and the honour of wearing epaulettes on his right shoulder. At the British Medical Association he was my chief for four years and I was devoted to him. The straightforward job specification for his life and work was loyalty to his country and to his profession. No wonder that as a personality he was tremendous.

Family celebration

SHOLTO FORMAN

VE Day was hot. Freakishly hot for May, and ironically hot for me. Had I not worked, slept, and eaten (not much else) for two and a half years in tropical heat, dreamt of cool cloudy days and Scotch rain, only to waken streaming with sweat as usual, to one more day of blistering sun and dusty toil?

Steaming through the Mediterranean it had been cold and rough, though the Rock was green, as only European springs are green, and many a war hardened eye on deck was as wet as my own as we moved in to berth and smelt the scents of Europe in May. We were not, by and large, a sentimental lot, but long suppressed emotions unexpectedly well up. England, we were warned, was exceptionally cold. As we steamed up the Irish Sea I dug out my European battledress from the bottom of my trunk; the thick hairy stuff was pleasantly reminiscent, and comfortable at sea. Travelling light from Liverpool, I packed off my tin trunk by train to Scotland, and set off for London with not much more than I wore on my back.

But the heat had preceded me, and as I walked out of Euston station I remember feeling as hot as I ever had in Asia; my hairy battledress was stirring up my prickly heat and scratching my neck like a wire brush. But who would be about in London on VE Day without his uniform? See the King and Churchill from the inside of some shrivelled wartime civvy suit? Not me. Anyway, I couldn't afford to buy one, so I stuck to my battledress. And it stuck to me.

Out of the hat

My clearest memory of the day was of sitting on a ledge high up on the Victoria Monument facing Buckingham Palace beside a Very

Important Person. We had been separated for two and a half years, linked only by fortnightly traffic in lettercards commenting on the world about us. Hers had been sensitive, humorous, sometimes infinitely sad, but of great moment to me, as I think mine were to her. They had helped to preserve my identity in a distant world which tended to convert one to an impersonal efficient machine, capable of keeping going in any conditions, with senses strictly suppressed. My sister was one of those rare beings with a gift for keeping families and friends together. She ran a sort of exchange in personal news, ideas, and changing philosophies, and trafficked in vignettes of those she was meeting and of familiar figures in our own circle of friends and the greater family. Her letters conveyed auras. So our meeting that day was a tremendous event. Besides, I had come straight to London to consult her on an important decision; but that is another story.

It would be unfair on the present generation to suggest that we cared more in those stricken years. But I remember a different intensity of caring; perhaps because of the common threat; perhaps because each meeting could so easily be the last, and sometimes was. I cared intensely about my sister; but caring was for everyone around you – the people you worked with, the people on the bus with you, the people in the bomb shelter. Caring was more vivid, stimulated perhaps by the appalling things that were happening to so many of them, and by the ordinary people around who were carrying on their dreary and wearying war jobs, having lost a husband, a child, all their possessions, sometimes all their family. It was a time when it was easy to love one's neighbour.

In action in Burma it was the same. You cursed your batman, the adjutant, your RAMC sergeant, and they, no doubt, you. A natural expression of frustration. We took risks for each other with equal lack of inhibitions that are searing to look back on. It was not, however, so easy to love one's enemy, and I don't remember putting much effort into that exercise. We cared intensely about winning the war, and winning it at any price we had to pay, believing that this held the only possible future for us and our like. Without being consciously jingoistic we cared intensely about Britain.

This was so for me in England in the early stages of the war at St Thomas's Hospital, and for my sister in MI5; so in raising an Indian casualty clearing station in south India, and in jungle training near Goa; so in action in Burma; and so in our exchange of letters, in a changing world where many of our contemporaries were dying. After two and a half years' separation the gods had selected this emotionally charged day to throw us together in the unlikely setting of a ledge on the Victoria Monument, at the very epicentre of the whole great war scene. A month's leave had come out of the blue, or rather out of the hat with my name on a slip of paper, under an agreeable scheme mysteriously labelled LIAP. It is the only time in my life I have been lucky in a raffle.

I cannot remember how we met before walking to Buckingham Palace, but I clearly remember how pale and how worn everyone looked in the streets. Either I had forgotten the appearance of London in wartime, or people had changed in the time I had been away. London was welcoming, but weary eyed, and there was little enough jubilation. The general sense was of relief, and of mutual warmth. Men stood me drinks before I could reach the bar. Women unexpectedly hugged me in the street. I felt ready to hug them all back and sometimes did. I hadn't seen any of them for two and a half years – years in another world which seemed half a lifetime to me.

The streets were full of people, walking, standing about, talking; there were no cars and few buses. Round Buckingham Palace the crowds steadily increased till they reached as far as I could see down the Mall, in the parks, and in Buckingham Palace Road – all solid with heads; and I was struck by the capacity of a crowd of such dimensions to manage itself without much police direction and without signs of disorder. I had got used to crowds in the far east.

After four decades recall must be inaccurate, but my memory is of a quiet crowd, with many families and children, in dull wartime dress, coloured up by patches of balloons and flags. When Churchill and the King appeared on the balcony the swaying sea of heads became a forest of arms, and the roar that went up was thunderous, prolonged, and insistently continuous. It was a chorus in unison that might have been orchestrated had it not been so obviously spontaneous. Churchill stood there in his characteristic stubby pugnacious form, making his V sign and beaming from ear to ear. And beside him the King. I remember feeling how this once shy and retiring man with a difficult stutter had grown into a leader of different but comparable stature to Winston.

The tremendous cheering and the constant reappearance of the Royal Family seemed to, and possibly did, continue for most of the blazing afternoon, each appearance seeming to become more relaxed and more personal, as the Queen and Princess Elizabeth and Princess Margaret joined the balcony party. I have never been greatly interested in ceremonial, but after absence in the far east, for years which were longer than their recorded calendar months, this was returning to a family celebration. I was a fully paid up member of the family, a piece of the crowd, and London was home, and I loved it.

A break in the clouds

But the pervading sense of relief in the final destruction of the Nazi menace was tempered. The Japs were still with us, and for those of us involved in their war VE Day was only a break in the clouds, a promise of fair weather. As I remember it, the current estimate of the cost of defeating the Japanese was three years and half a million lives. For me, as for tens of thousands of others, the war started again at the end of leave. I was due to sail for Bombay in a month and could expect exile for three years (some said seven before repatriation); that is for those of us who survived. Tomorrow I was to meet the girl I knew I loved. But was it zany to think of marriage at this state of the game? Anyway, how would we find each other? We had known each other for six months before I left, separated in different parts of England for three of them. Letters are one thing, but how would it be?

Born a cautious Scot and analytical by training, the demand for instant decision on this far reaching matter put all my concepts to the test. For it has always gone against my grain to be pushed into action before the instinctive time for decision arrives. I felt no affection for the Japanese that day. But if hopes had been dupes, fears turned out to be resounding liars. We were married at three days' notice in the kirk I had been christened in at Beattock in Dumfrieshire, amid all my family but one – a brother confined to hospital – by the superb organisation of my available brothers and sisters, on a quantity of hoarded champagne, and, I suspect, slightly black market fare.

We went fishing in the highlands and my wife caught more trout than I, a long experienced rod, could bring to net. I incurred her wrath for the first time by standing her up in the Station Hotel lounge in Morar while forgetfully drinking whisky with our ghillie, a man so greatly after my own heart as to bring me to do so dreadful a thing to my bride. He was, I think, a chief petty officer RN on leave in his own village. Back eventually to Brown's Hotel in Dover Street, where five days' stay in discreet luxury, plus a massive reception for half St Thomas's Hospital and a fair slice of MI5, cost me the crippling sum of £77.

We'll meet again

I boarded the trooper and my wife went back to run her surgical ward at St Thomas's, and we reckoned, looking on the bright side, that we should meet again in three years. I gathered up the reins as resident medical officer, No 5 Commando near Poona, and the sound of machine guns on exercise fired the most chilling reflex associations down my spine I can remember.

But fears were liars again. The bombs on Hiroshima and Nagasaki were dropped as we were packing an exhausted looking tramp steamer in Bombay harbour for the invasion of Penang Island. None of us wept for the victims. Perhaps we were wrong, but on the night the war ended I don't think any of us gave a damn. Reprieve is sweet. I was home six months later. VJ Day felt a bit of an anticlimax, and the ensuing "Festival of Britain" distinctly out of joint with the times. Nobody felt festive, just glad to be alive and unharrassed.

My wife and I lived happily ever after. But I still have a compulsive habit of touching wood.

Poor substitute for real life

RONALD GIBSON

I cannot particularly remember VE Day. I was in the wilds of what had been called Italian Somaliland (the scene of the first and, for a long time, only triumph of the Allied forces) in my fourth year overseas, being responsible for the health of the territory in general and the reduction of the appalling VD rate in particular. VE Day meant that one day I would be able to go home again and be reunited with my family – whereas if the Germans had won I suppose we might never have met again; and at least I was still alive and in one piece.

Looking back on those days to VE Day and beyond it is extraordinary how one never really lived. They were exciting at times, enjoyable, and different, yet they represented an insecure and unnatural existence and a poor substitute for the real and fulfilling life one had expected after qualification.

VE Day somehow seemed to bring this home with a bang. There was a sudden realisation of how tired one was of it all and an irresistible longing to have done with it. Moreover, there still remained the worry of what was to happen to those of us who were far from home now it was "all over". The change from war to peace could well be a disturbing and traumatic anticlimax. And it was.

Letters from home

My wife had written to me practically every day since I had left her in Cornwall, at 24 hours' notice, for an unknown destination. It was snowing, our four year old daughter had pneumonia, and the baby whooping cough. I had a travel warrant to Glasgow and some sandwiches provided by the mess cook; she had to pack up and

73

journey back to Hampshire in our clapped out old car. I kept all her letters (and she kept mine). Reading them again has been a pretty emotional experience.

The families we left behind had a much worse time than some of us overseas and I am appalled today at the way in which I appeared to treat so lightly her description of the crises she had to cope with alone, summed up by the comment, "This confounded war seems to be eternal. I suppose one day we shall be all together again." She didn't even know where I was when she wrote that.

Clearly, I had the impression that because I was overseas I was the one making all the sacrifices and she really ought not to grumble about such minor troubles as having to look after a family in wartime; no home of her own and no husband; air raids and flying bombs; the blackout and a shortage of food – after all, she was in England.

The long, anxious days came to an end with D Day. At last something was happening and even those first uncertain months after the landings served to underline the relief and excitement now that the days of waiting were over and we were on the move. It is unexpected therefore to read that she found it difficult, when VE Day came, to raise any other emotion than one of profound relief. No jubilant rejoicing nor sense of triumph. Even the sound of the church bells left her surprisingly (and uncharacteristically) unmoved. In the last paragraph of this particular letter she says, "Now it is all over, I wonder what the future holds for us all." Even today, 40 years on, these letters are difficult to read without a nasty, hurt feeling inside.

Picking up the pieces

A month or so after VE Day I drew four weeks' LIAP leave. I left everything (including a Siamese cat, never to be seen again) at a moment's notice, thinking I would be home in a few days. I jumped on to a little Dutch ship bouncing up and down in Mogadiscio harbour. The master invited me to "Schnapps and Whitbreads, isn't it?" in his cabin and we journeyed slowly to Mombasa (the wrong direction for me). After a seemingly endless and expensive stay in an hotel I was off by ship again, this time to Cairo, and then – after more weeks of waiting – to Glasgow in convoy.

By now I had realised that there was little priority available for personnel going on leave.

Betty, as soon as she heard of my impending return, had summarily evicted our unwanted lodgers and busied herself trying to make the home we hadn't seen for over five years look as though we had never left it (including two cats and a dog).

We met on neutral territory in a Southampton hotel, where she embarrassed us both by failing to remember whether or not I took sugar in my coffee. Our younger daughter – by then aged 4 – had decided to call me "Hickler" because he was the only man she had ever heard of (though, thank goodness, she hadn't seen him) and even gifts of apparently very acceptable presents from this strange man she had to call "Daddy" failed to wheedle him into her affections for a long time.

I spent the month working hard, trying to pick up the pieces of my small and very broken down practice (which had only known me for about 18 months before I joined up) but, even though I had only a month or two to go before eventual demobilisation, no amount of pleading persuaded the War Office to let me stay longer. I shall never forget the dreadful anticlimax of having to return overseas again after that brief glimpse of home and family. I endured a Mediterranean cruise (during which I heard of the atomic bombs dropped on Japan), another long stay in Cairo, and a flight down Africa in a shaky Dakota long overdue for the scrapyard – as witness the elegant crash landing on leaving Wadi-Halfa.

I protested strongly at the proposal that I should now go to British Somaliland, and, as a result, was given a disbanding field ambulance to command while I waited for my demob papers. Meanwhile my practice and newly acquainted family were left once again in frustrated suspense.

Eventualy I flew back to Cairo (in another Dakota – what wonderful machines they were), journeyed to Alexandria by train, across the Mediterranean by sea to Toulon and then across France to Dieppe, Folkestone, and an army issue civilian suit. It all took weeks.

I think we can be forgiven for not particularly remembering VE Day, yet it is unbelievable to think that it could have seemed to be just another day. After six years as a number (133953) I now had a name again and could make my own decisions (right or wrong). There was freedom to come and go wherever and whenever I wanted, and the joy of my own family to greet in the morning.

I suppose it comes under the heading of "redemption through suffering" but thank goodness Betty needn't have worried about our future. Family life and family doctoring have made it all very worth while – thanks to VE Day.

Journey's end

ARNOLD GOUREVITCH

It was Monday 7 May. It was in the officers' mess. We were a field surgical unit stuck on to a field dressing station. We had arrived in Trieste, capital of a province with the lovely name Venezia-Julia. Someone switched on the wireless and we heard General Alexander say something about millions of Germans laying down their arms, which seemed a very unGermanlike thing to do. We knew they were in a bad way because we had seen their convoys – some of their vehicles drawn by horses.

We listened to the voice on the radio in that semi-cynical half believing way. Then it dawned on us that perhaps we had really won – perhaps the war was over. At that moment a signal arrived addressed to me; it was my "python" notification. I had no idea what "python" stood for but I knew what it meant: it meant home after three and a half years overseas. Almost on the instant I shouted to the lad behind the bar, "Twenty two double whiskies!" It was a reflex, like a western sheriff shouting, "Drinks on the house!". The whiskies appeared and we consumed them quietly; it hadn't really sunk in. The next thing that happened was odd to say the least. We formed ourselves into a gigantic rugger scrum using a wastepaper basket as a ball, and for the next 20 minutes we fought like tigers for possession of that basket. We then flung ourselves down exhausted in a giggly stupefied state – it still hadn't sunk in.

Looking for the war

It was in fact the end of a journey which had begun long before – indeed for me when I joined the TA before the war. I joined because I felt sure there would be a war.

Once it happened I was delighted to cast off the trappings of

77

"Civvy Street" and join my mates in a TA field ambulance. I was introduced to the chaos and confusion of war in France in 1940. I was also privileged throughout the war to meet some good men who stood out from their fellows. These exceptional men all had one thing in common: they were calm while the storm raged about them. One was my orderly, Quinlan. I remember him counting the bombs 1–6 leaving a German aircraft while I cowered under an ambulance.

France was followed by a strange lull; where was the war, I asked. Someone testily said, "In the middle east". This sounded promising and I said as much. Another older colleague said, "I suppose you see yourself roaming the desert on a white horse waving a sword". Not a bad idea, I thought.

After a 10-week sea voyage round the Cape escorted by an ancient battleship – *Ramilles* – we arrived in Port Tewfik, and the desert sand looked like snow in the moonlight. I have a vivid memory of our troops marching through the streets of Cairo wearing Bombay bloomers. These were shorts turned up and buttoned and they still came below the knee. The effect on the local citizenry of an RAMC unit thus attired on the march may be imagined. Their money was on Rommel.

In and out of the bag

We went to Crete. The German airborne invasion duly took place. Our hospital, No 7 General, was on a nice level bit of ground by the sea. The German paratroops must have liked the look of it because they dropped on it after a preliminary softening up.

I was having a morning dip in the briny with a charming New Zealand surgeon called Christie. We saw no reason to come ashore and so we remained in the ocean, total equipment a couple of tin hats. Christie had just come out of Greece and was well informed on the various types of German aircraft and so gave me a short tutorial.

The New Zealanders eventually drove out the paratroops and we shifted the wounded to some caves which gave some protection. But the end became inevitable and we wended our way south over the mountains down towards Sphakia, the point of evacuation which I never actually saw. I was placed in charge of the wounded and the remnants of our unit. The boys carried the wounded up the steep gullies on doors torn off a church, whence they were conveyed by German trucks back to our old hospital area, except that now it was a large prison camp containing 8000 men.

The next six months were not altogether unpleasant – indeed I learned many things, one being that I was determined not to remain an unwilling guest indefinitely.

The last batch of prisoners was due for transfer to the mainland and thence to Germany. We decided it was time to go – "we" being "Skipper" Dorney, an Australian medical officer, and myself. I can still remember the awful twanging noise he made climbing over the wire, while I waited, knowing I was to be next.

Then followed a spell of six months' wandering round the lovely mountainous island of Crete in the company of various mates. I cannot speak highly enough of the hospitality and courage of our Cretan hosts, and I must record my gratitude to Georgios Karvounakis, the dentist who took us into his home on our first night out of camp. I rang the bell of his house – it was in a square in Chania not unlike Tavistock Square but much smaller, and opposite was the German "Feldkommandatur" – and a maid answered the ring. She was dressed in a lace cap and apron and gave a squeak of apprehension as she looked at two scruffy looking men grinning reassuringly at her. From the depths of the house came a strong voice, that of Georgios Karvounakis: "Come in, sit down, make yourselves at home". That phrase has the power of Holy Writ for me. Georgios Karvounakis gave us hospitality, a night's rest, clothes, and a start. He knew perfectly well the risk he was taking when he welcomed us into his home. The following day – that is, the day we left – some German officers arrived and billeted themselves in Georgios's home, remaining there for many months.

Then it was back to the middle east, this time with a field surgical unit (No 8) in the company of my old friend the late Bob Cope – a journey which started in the Nile Delta, continued via the western desert, north Africa, and Sicily into Italy. Once again we were looking for the war.

I began to live again when we joined the New Zealand division whom I had last met in Crete. Big bronzed men with the black and white New Zealand flash on their shoulders. I have to say that I think the world of the New Zealanders. I will always have a soft spot for them and we in the UK should never forget their contribution.

Even they couldn't crack the German 1st Parachute Division at Cassino in Italy. I saw Monastery Hill like 5 November lit by incessant shellfire. The 1st Paras, having gone to ground, laughed at this and popped up next morning as chirpy as ever. They were superb troops.

Our field surgical unit was with the advanced dressing station of a New Zealand field ambulance. Someone had the idea that we should hold seriously wounded casualties forward, because advancing tanks might block the evacuation route. Perhaps they were right, I don't know. Helicopters hadn't been invented. I learned then that wounded men do not do well within sight and sound of shellfire. I remember sitting on the bed of a soldier with a gunshot belly wound. There was a loud bang and I saw his pupils dilate with fear. I remember thinking this was no place for him.

After the second and third battles of Cassino I was ordered back to Sicily and said a fond farewell to the kiwis, whom I shall never forget. I extracted a promise from Harold Edwards, consultant surgeon at Fifth Army Group in Naples that he would not let me languish in Sicily. He was as good as his word. I joined 10 FSU in the hills south of Bologna.

Soon afterwards we joined an American field hospital. This was an experience in itself. The Americans had nightly movies. I remember the following exchange between two GIs: "Say, who's Lauren Bacall?" "Oh, you know she's that tall slinky gal." A gentleman called Joe Finegold won everyone's money at a crap game and then had the nerve to be posted. As he was waiting for the ambulance to take him to his new unit a friend shouted, "Hey, get this guy an ambulance, he'll buy one".

Ready to go home

I had never particularly wanted to go home from the day war was declared and indeed only had two short weekend "leaves" between the fall of France and departure to the middle east. Home meant nothing to me. I simply cannot explain the feeling. I just wanted to go to the war wherever it was for as long as it lasted. But from the moment it finished the army had no further meaning and I wanted to get out.

I had no expectations – that is, no job waiting for me. I wanted to see my mother and father and my sister, whom I adored, and to get stuck into the business of becoming a surgeon in peacetime, though I had no idea what that entailed.

We had arrived in a little village called Cervignano just outside

Trieste after a long trip and a long slog up Italy (what a lovely country it was, even though devastated by war). I had never consciously moved forward during the whole of the war until our advance northwards across the Po Valley. My war had been marked by retreats and hurried evacuations; I had been a POW. Now here we were in Trieste.

Tito's partisans shambled about the streets in small platoons, vaguely hostile, unkempt, their rifles and equipment dirty and uncared for. The New Zealanders regarded them as frankly hostile and put themselves in a defensive posture, Bren guns facing outwards. They were taking no chances. What little conversation I had had with the troops convinced me that a government of the people by the people was coming. It was all a case of, "What I expect to receive when I get home". No one mentioned work – this was definitely a dirty word.

Consulting my diary I find a menu dated 8 May 1945. Apparently we had what was called "A Victory Dinner". We undoubtedly enjoyed it. It was I am sure hilarious. I cannot remember it.

When in Bologna, which I knew was renowned for its silk materials, I had bought 30 pairs of silk stockings and six silk pram covers, because my sister was due to have a baby and these seemed appropriate. The thing was to get there before the Americans, because once they were there the prices rocketed.

I arrived at New Street station in Birmingham. There on the platform was my sister, heavy with child, and my parents.

I don't remember

CHARLES HILL

The awful truth is that I can remember little about VE Day – indeed my recollection of Armistice Day nearly 66 years ago is brighter. Maybe this is due to the fact that my wife was producing our fifth child at the time. Then again, as every geriatric knows, the memory of what happened years ago is easier than the recall of the events of yesterday. I do fairly recollect, however, that there was on that day a meeting between representatives of the royal colleges and the BMA on some subject relating to a national health service. What the subject was escapes me, though I can remember the vigour of Alfred Webb-Johnson and the silence of Lord Moran at that meeting. But we certainly proceeded with it with scarcely a reference to the great event of the day; perhaps we were anaesthetised by the low key discussions with Henry Willink. Certainly we had no idea that the forthcoming general election would mean that he would be replaced by Aneurin Bevan, and that tranquillity would give way to turmoil.

Maybe the victory so confidently expected was taken for granted. Possibly my generation recalled the appalling problems which confronted our country in the years that followed the Armistice of 1918. I just do not know. But I do know that my dimness of recollection is not due to excessive libation on that great day ... No, I cannot remember.

New thinking and actions

JAMES HOWIE

For two years before VE Day I served as a deputy assistant director of pathology in the War Office in London – a very minor post but one that brought a most interesting range of duties and contacts. For two years before that I had the good fortune to serve as a pathologist in Nigeria, where we had an important preoccupation with the danger that yellow fever might be exported to Egypt and India via the air route through west Africa – the only quick way from London after 1940, when the Mediterranean route was closed, until the Allied victory in north Africa in May 1943.

The end of London's war

I remember VE Day in London very well; but a more emotional recollection is of what was for us in London the real end of the war.

Two weeks before VE Day, on 24 April, the Speaker switched on the lantern light in the tower of the House of Commons. It had been switched off during the blackout, but with the capture of the last of the V1 and V2 sites it was judged that the end of the war would not now be long delayed and, as a symbol of the successful defence of freedom, the lantern light could be switched on again. As dusk approached a smallish crowd collected in Parliament Square. The Speaker explained what he was about to do, and what his action symbolised. Then he said in a level and modest but moving way: "I now switch on our lantern 'light'". It was so effective and so English (I mean English) that the crowd's response was at first subdued, but gradually rose to a proper cheer. Strangers greeted each other with handshakes and embraces and a real but quiet sense of gratitude that we had survived. For me, that was the end of London's war; and a very moving moment it was.

VE Day was something different – not really an anticlimax but something a bit less wildly enthusiastic and spontaneous than Armistice Day at 11 am on 11 November 1918, when it seemed that the first world war suddenly rushed to a surprising end and people went mad with joy and relief. I was an 11 year old then, at school in Aberdeen, but I still recall the ecstatic joy and our headmaster's calling the school together to declare a holiday, and to urge restraint in our rejoicing out of consideration for the many who had their dead to remember.

The end of fighting in Europe in 1945 had been creeping up on us for some weeks, and we still had the war in the far east to finish. That seemed likely to be a long and desperate affair – we did not know then about nuclear weapons. VE Day dawned bright, warm, and clear. There was a generally cheerful but fairly restrained gathering of crowds at strategic places in London. I was in Whitehall when Winston Churchill appeared with colleagues on the balcony of the old Ministry of Health to announce the signing of the armistice, and he was loudly and gratefully cheered. But that was not the only note. Near me was a critical group of men who cheered with the rest of us, but then murmured among themselves. "Well, we've won his bloody war for him and his Tories; what'll he do for us?" "You have a bloody hope," came the reply. My own hopes, which I did not express, were that Winston would not sell out to the right wing Tories but go for the middle ground, using his unique reputation and deserved fame to maintain the wartime spirit of national unity. Perhaps that was a naive hope; certainly his first election addresses quickly killed it off. But on VE Day we did not yet know what was to follow.

I was in the evening crowd outside Buckingham Palace to hear the King's broadcast and cheer the party on the balcony. His courage in making his speech, which was firm and clear, and his bearing throughout the war, and that of his Queen and the princesses, quite clearly went to all hearts. The crowds in the Mall were the happiest I saw that day, and they were quite unequivocally royalist. Crossing Vauxhall Bridge on my way back to the RAMC headquarters mess in Millbank I was moved by the skilful floodlighting of St Paul's and of the Inns of Court. This battered city still stood and we wished for a new beginning – perhaps our thinking was too wishful. The evening paper was sold behind a billboard on which was chalked, "Germans say they'll be our allies in 20 years".

Different priorities

Regarding the previous two years in the War Office, there was much to reflect upon. I recalled our part in fostering the tremendous work that went into learning enough about how to use penicillin and blood transfusion as near the front line as possible. The names of Florey and Cairns, and of Whitby, Boyd, and Buttle shone through that memory. In fact, surgeons who served in both the 1914–18 war and in that of 1939–45 paid the real tribute to the success of the policy of penicillin for all wounded, early blood transfusion, and rapid evacuation to base. These surgeons testified that they would not have believed it possible that wounds could be so clean or men so soon able to stand major surgery. Organising enough supplies of penicillin and blood was a perpetual struggle; but the logistics of having them available right forward were continually calling for new thinking and actions. I recalled how, near the end of May 1944, as D Day approached, it seemed that we could not hope to get first aid boxes with penicillin, brief and clear instructions, and yellow identifying labels ready for the first wave of landing craft. In our branch all of us, except the general and his assistant director, dropped everything else and organised ourselves into a team of packers with a process line to get the boxes ready in sufficient numbers. My part was to make the final check to ensure that the contents were complete and to affix the yellow labels. It was an interesting industrial experience – not at all boring, for we had cheerful conversation from a very mixed company. At the end of it we all felt pleasantly relaxed; but by evening my yellow vision was so overused and so exhausted that I continually got into trouble through being unable to tell the white from the yellow ball at snooker.

On VE Day I recalled how worth while our efforts had been. I reflected sadly that we had never been able to secure a real, operational, priority for penicillin production in Britain to grow as quickly as could have been possible. We secured only "paper priority" – permission for pharmaceutical firms to engage labour and erect laboratories – but there were no men and no materials to be had. Later, about the end of 1944, we secured real operational priority to manufacture a scrub typhus vaccine, about whose value we were totally unconvinced, but which was demanded on the grounds that it would help the morale of troops destined for jungle warfare. Operation "Tyburn" (typhus vaccine needed in a helluva hurry, as I explained to the bright young man who produced the code name) really was given a true priority. But atomic bombs made the jungle warfare unnecessary, and chloramphenicol knocked out the scrub typhus so effectively that the vaccinated rubber planters who went back to Malaya when it was regained provided no evidence as to whether the vaccine worked or not.

Waste of precious life

On VE Day the recollection of the death of one particular friend and colleague focused my feelings of grief for all the terrible losses and waste of good effort. My friend was Dr E C (Ted) Smith, a Dublin microbiologist, who was medical director of the Medical Research Laboratory outside Lagos. He served the medical war effort in Nigeria in countless unselfish ways; and he knew his tropical microbiology with a sure instinct for what mattered, and with a fund of information going back to the final convincing sad proof that yellow fever was indeed caused by a virus and not by Noguchi's leptospire. Smith was present at the deaths of Stokes and Noguchi; and it was Smith who backed up and urged acceptance of the idea of a field test to discover, against the odds, if vaccine might be used to make the west African airfields into genuinely yellow fever free zones. What I personally, and many others, owed to Ted Smith in the period 1941–3 is beyond telling in detail. He had been due for home leave in 1939 but declined to go for two reasons: he thought that the 18 month limit for a tour in Nigeria was total nonsense (the nuns at the convent knew that too); and he confessed to a presentiment that he would lose his life at sea. He resisted all pressures to take home leave until the summer of 1943, by which time the victory in north Africa had greatly reduced the risk to convoys from submarine warfare. I had returned home in April 1943, and met him in London before he left to return to Nigeria. He was still unhappy, and with good cause: on the voyage to Freetown a lone raider dropped a bomb down the funnel of his ship, and Smith's cabin was exactly where the bomb exploded. For me personally the sadness of that particular waste of a precious life was overwhelming.

*   *   *

I am happy to contribute these thoughts in affectionate memory of Elston, a friendly colleague and a military gentleman in the best sense.

Its real importance

LIPMANN KESSEL

I am sure that the full significance of VE Day did not really strike me at the time. A few days later, however, its importance came home with full force.

I was quietly working as a surgeon in a general hospital in Celle, West Germany. It was, I think, 6 General Hospital, but I can't be sure. It was under the command of a Colonel Day, RAMC, whom I had previously met as the commanding officer of a CCS in Tunisia, which was a long time ago in those days.

Tunis to Taranto

I had arrived in north Africa as a replacement surgeon for Charles Rob, who had been injured on his first parachute drop as surgeon in charge of the first surgical team of 16 Para Field Ambulance. I think he had broken his ankle on landing, and I was sent to replace him.

We had a short, sharp battle outside Tunis before the First and Eighth Armies joined finally to eradicate the German presence in north Africa. We then went off to Sidi bel Abbes, of Foreign Legion fame, to train for the next campaign. This was to be a short trip into Sicily, where our brigade was to take and secure the bridge across the Gornalunga River by dropping in the Plain of Catania. The campaign was successful, and there were more casualties from malaria than gunshot wounds. We spent only five days in Sicily before returning to our base in Tunisia.

From Tunis we set out by ship to Taranto in the toe of Italy, and worked our way north with the famous Popski and his private army, chasing the retreating Germans up Italy, which finally collapsed on account of the Italian uprising.

We were then sent back to Britain to prepare for the western thrust into Europe. We prepared for one battle after another, and I think we were briefed for no less than 16 campaigns, of which 15 were cancelled, before we set out one sunny Sunday morning to take the northernmost bridge cross the Rhine. The now famous Battle of Arnhem followed. Arnhem was a splendid failure, characterised by the great contrast between the ineptitude of those who planned the operation and the bravery of the troops who fought in it. I was in the bag for a short weekend only, but it took me nearly five months in occupied Holland before I was able to return across the Rhine by canoe to our own troops.

The full significance

After a short rest I asked to go back to Germany, in the hope of being present at the final victory. I was posted as a surgeon to a British general hospital. It so happened that we were in the area held by the Guards Armoured Division, whose medical services were under the control of the legendary Glyn Hughes. He had received a message under a white flag from the opposite German command: typhus had broken out and an epidemic was feared. Glyn Hughes asked me to go in with an RAMC squad under the shield of a battalion of the Guards Armoured Division.

It was about this time that the formal surrender was accepted by Montgomery on Lüneburg Heath. More or less at the same time I found myself in the Belsen concentration camp. The other medical group was an MRC nutrition unit led by Dr (now Dame) Janet Vaughan, who suffered much by what she had seen in the ghastliness of this louse ridden remnant of an extermination camp. I recall that I picked up a book lying alongside a dead inmate. This was a copy of the *Contes Drolatiques* by Voltaire.

I have recently looked at this book again and I see inscribed in the flyleaf the following words: "I picked up this book at Belsen Bergen concentration camp, in a hut measuring 8ft × 6ft and filled with dead and near dead victims. The book was covered in DDT – the flower of European culture covered in anti-louse powder".

I think it might have been at that moment that the full historical and human significance of VE Day came upon me, and has remained with me throughout my life.

Exigencies of war

HEBER LANGSTON

Park Prewett Hospital, Basingstoke, a major mental hospital administered by Hampshire County Council, was a large rambling block of Edwardian buildings in extensive grounds, some four miles north of the then small market town. Early in the second world war it was taken over by the Emergency Medical Service, all its patients being evacuated to Scotland, but leaving behind an administration staff used to a quiet, slow moving, orderly life who never became fully accustomed to running an emergency hospital in the stress conditions of war.

Invasion from London

Imported into this quiet hospital there arrived large secondments of nursing staff from the London teaching hospitals, St Thomas's, St Mary's, and the Westminster, with separate deputy matrons, resident junior medical staff, and visiting consultants from the same hospitals still working part time in London and fitting in visits as and when they could, with a few – such as myself – who still had unavoidable major commitments at other special hospitals. In spite of such varying backgrounds and unpredictable visiting times (one St Mary's surgeon always visited at night, operating from 10 pm until the early hours, and demanding a cooked breakfast before he left in the dark or grey light of morning), a common unity of purpose, service, and esprit de corps did develop as all became acclimatised to the exigencies of war – disturbed only by the occasional visits of imperious matrons from parent hospitals, visiting service chiefs, and EMS consultant advisers, some with impossible demands which were complied with, sidetracked or conveniently forgotten, as circumstances demanded. Portering, theatre, and plaster technicians were provided by RAMC orderlies – seldom of high calibre, since the best of that corps were seldom left permanently in Britain.

Initially the patients were derived from London and the vulnerable coast cities of Portsmouth and Southampton but as D Day approached virtually all these patients were transferred to "safe" hospitals elsewhere, as Park Prewett became designated the major hospital for D Day casualties returned to Britain.

Care of the wounded

On the first night after the landings a train containing approximately 300 casualties arrived at a nearby railway siding. Staff duties had been previously designated, consultant and junior medical being divided into three rotating groups of three teams each, the first group to "triage", the second to operative and other acute emergency work, and the third to ward assessment, observation, and record initiation.

Our instructions were that those seconded to initial assessment and examination were to admit only those who required urgent treatment or close observation or who were moribund. This was achieved by a system of colour labelling – red, yellow, and purple for those admitted, and green for onward transfer. For this operation we were allowed one and a half hours, during which time the train was "turned around" and reloaded with those fit for onward transfer.

Casualties were unloaded from ambulances at the entrance to an empty storage shed on to trolleys moved up marked out lines to respective awaiting teams consisting of a consultant, houseman, two orderlies, and a nurse. All arrived as they had fallen in battle, fully clothed, muddy, blood stained, some with simple splinting of limbs. An orderly stripped off clothing as necessary. Examination of exhausted, sometimes seasick, soldiers varying in consciousness was often difficult. The blood staining over an open would could so easily overshadow a potentially much more dangerous chest or abdominal injury, with a hidden entrance wound and confusing or minimal physical signs, whilst all the while the examining surgeon might be aware of a lengthening queue moving towards him.

Operating by the second team began about 2 pm as soon as an anaesthetist thought practicable, a junior assessing priorities. The operating theatres were far from ideal, being converted wash-houses in which prewar mental patients had apparently been showered once a week. Cramped, none too adequately equipped, and, in the early days, sometimes with a second table fitted in to speed up procedures. Those selected for operation would, of course, be further examined in the theatre and I recollect deciding that a laparotomy was necessary and finding – in a patient sent to me because of a bullet shattered femur – a severe bladder injury as well (an alarming discovery for an orthopaedic surgeon some years removed from his general surgical training).

Time consuming radiological examinations were avoided as far as possible, especially since, although the theatre was equipped with a portable x ray machine, developing facilities were so far away that it necessitated the radiographer bicycling in total darkness to another building some distance away along a winding path, and returning the same way with developed plates in their holders on her handlebars. On one occasion, after an exceptionally long absence, a search party found the unfortunate girl in a neglected rose bed with her bicycle and the plates on top of her, having herself sustained an ankle injury. It is not recollected if the plates were thereafter of any great assistance.

Children and civilians

Apart from this EMS work, I had also been retained in civilian service because I happened to be the only remaining active surgeon on the staff of a 350 bed children's orthopaedic hospital, some 12 miles distant from Park Prewett. Inevitably sleep was somewhat short in the early post D Day weeks; but at that hospital, where there were also two other whole time residents, it was possible to carry out one operating session per week and to visit as time allowed scattered county outpatient orthopaedic clinics, particularly in Southampton – where I was then attached as a temporary visiting consultant – as there were some civilian casualties to be treated, although fortunately these had greatly diminished as the result of the crippling of the German air force before D Day arrived.

When VE Day itself came this most interesting, hard worked, and exhausting period of my wartime life was already over; but two contrasting memories of its two phases remain: first, of the grim sight of weary families trudging out of Southampton in the late afternoon to sleep in church halls and elsewhere in the days of the blitz; and, second, of the dawn chorus as I drove home along country lanes from Park Prewett in the early hours of a summer morning shortly after D Day.

*　　*　　*

Finally, a word about Elston Grey-Turner who, although I did not get to know him until the early 1950s, became a very firm friend, loyal confidant and shrewd adviser when he became secretary of the central committee for hospital medical services for several years during the middle years of my chairmanship – a time of some tensions and difficult decisions during which, on the one hand, we were striving to obtain a fuller recognition by established consultants as their negotiating body within the National Health Service and a greater share with the royal colleges in policy making, so that the CCHMS should become the initiator of policy within the joint consultants committee; and to be recognised as speaking with authority for all consultants in negotiations with the review body. Much of our success in all these fields is owed to the wise counsel of Elston and the path was often made so much easier by his dry caustic humour and wit.

Why I missed it

BERNARD LENNOX

I should be disqualified from this line up on at least two counts: first, that I never had the pleasure of meeting Grey-Turner (though his father, Sir George, was my chief as a student at Newcastle, and a very senior colleague later at Hammersmith); and second, that I missed VE Day altogether – wasn't there and didn't know it had happened. This will therefore have to be largely an explanation for the latter statement.

I was called to the colours in March 1940, from a very junior academic post in pathology, and sent straight out to Singapore. There I spent 18 months in all but peacetime conditions as regimental MO to three battalions of Gunners, including the famous coast defence guns that were unjustly accused of pointing the wrong way (it was the Japanese who most unfairly arrived by the wrong way). For two hectic months of war in Malaya I was pathologist and general dogsbody to 1 Malaya General Hospital. Then, of course, in the bag, into Changi again as a POW.

That was hectic, too, for some months, but the story has been told often enough. I had the good fortune to prove at necropsy that an epidemic apparently of infective encephalitis was in fact Wernicke's (cerebral beri-beri), which saved quite a few lives, formed a basis for detailed study of that previously elusive entity by the strong group of physicians who were there, and, incidentally, saw me safely into a most suitable job after the war. The sick died or (mostly) recovered, most of the fit combatants were sent up to Siam to build the Siam–Burma railway of evil memory, and Changi became a relatively peaceful place, if semi-starved.

Worst part of captivity

In mid-1943 a group of 30 MOs and 200 (mostly RAMC) other

93

ranks were sent up to Siam (K force, to be followed by a smaller group called L force). We found we were to look after civilian conscripts who had been sent up from Malaya to work on the railway. Not much is heard of them, but there were probably as many of them (Malays, Chinese, and Tamils mostly) as there were POWs, and though they were in intent treated better than our own people they were exposed to much the same conditions, had no corporate discipline of their own, and had no medical personnel, so that their sickness and death rates could well have been worse than ours. I know no official figures.

With three RAMC privates and a Gunner sergeant I went up river by barge 200 kilometres from base to a Japanese hospital established near the line of the railway. We helped to build a most primitive "hospital" of attap thatched roof over bare earth, in monsoon conditions, and soon acquired our first patients. Starvation, malaria, dysentery, and tropical ulcer were the rule – often all four together – and food and drugs were all grossly deficient. I was joined by another MO from the Malayan Civil Service, but even with his greater experience there was little we could do. We had in all through our hands about 400 patients, and discharged only 60 of them alive. At least the clothes of the dead, such as they were, gave us something to dress others with.

That was for me by far the worst part of captivity – of my life, for that matter – and most of K force had similar tales to tell: three died, all working alone with no other MO to deal with their own illnesses.

Various odd jobs

Things were a good deal better after the railway was finished, and the combination of supply difficulties with intense pressure to open the supply route (for assault from Burma on India) that lay at the root of the whole tragic affair no longer applied. Our survivors were sent down to base. I travelled up and down the railway on various odd jobs for some months: addition to the Malay learnt in Singapore of a smattering of Japanese made me a useful communication link. A spell in Burma in the monsoon season was an eye opener as to what real rain can be like.

The chronic sick survivors of our Malayan patients were gathered into large hospital camps near the base of the railway at Kamburi, a prosperous town with abundant food supplies. K and

L forces gathered mostly in one such camp. We included when gathered together a substantial range of medical skills; food was much better, and medical supplies also. My microscope had packed up and I was no longer any use as a pathologist, but I was the nearest approach to an interpreter that we had. Discovery of a bottle of white powder in the Japanese dispensary with a name ending in "cain" led to my becoming a spinal anaesthetist: over 400 spinals without a death is my proud record. Nearly all were for tropical ulcer, for which excision was the only effective treatment; 50 required amputation. Two of us also ran an isolation ward for a cholera epidemic; under the conditions a 50% death rate was not unreasonable. It was – as often with cholera – a thinly disguised blessing: the authorities reacted vigorously, sanitation improved, and the death rate from gut infections generally fell rapidly.

A sustaining luxury at this time was news. There was an English language newspaper still, surprisingly, being printed in Siam, and copies often reached us. It told, of course, only of sweeping Japanese victories, but it was encouraging to note that each Allied disaster occurred a little nearer Japan (or Berlin) than the last.

Little except anxieties

By early 1945 the work was done and the hospital camp disbanded. We were returned to normal POW camps. We found that combatant officers had been removed to separate camps, and the medicals were almost the only officers left. It was a time of little activity, and I remember little except anxieties. The Axis seemed to be crumbling, but news was now rare and scarcely better than rumour. If the Burma campaign carried on into Siam, what might not happen to us? Even if, as was more likely, the Japs retreating from Burma were simply cut off from Japan and left to their own devices, we might find ourselves hostages or worse. Such are the effects of inactivity – up to that time most of us had been busy enough to limit our worrying to day by day affairs.

In this state, without knowing it, we spent VE Day.

A Siamese contractor delivering food to the camp contrived to pass the news of German capitulation about 10 days later, neatly done under the noses of guards at considerable risk to himself. We rejoiced, naturally: all resources were mustered for a grand celebratory concert, and some enormous cakes were baked, of rice laced with various minor luxuries, and decorated with Union Jack designs in mercurochrome and methylene blue. It was marvellous of course, but the problem remained: how long would the Japanese hold out, and what would happen to us?

Fortunately for me inactivity did not last long. I went back up the railway with an Anglo-Australian party to a wood cutting camp in dense jungle (the railway burned wood) to join a large Dutch party with two Dutch MOs. It was a pleasant enough spot, with only the size of the attached cemetery to remind one how much the railway had cost to build. An intelligent Australian sergeant had a manic spell and we had a distracting fortnight keeping him out of trouble. One of the Dutch MOs maintained that the north to south travel of the sun was linear against my own insistence of a sine curve: we set up a 10 foot high bamboo sundial to test this by noon measurements of the shadow. But, alas, the experiment was interrupted by a summons for the whole party to be moved back down to base.

Nothing unusual about this. We arrived at Kamburi and the train halted outside a large POW camp. Over it flags were flying, mostly Union Jacks and one Dutch. Our captors quietly vanished. I had missed VJ Day too: Hiroshima had happened 10 days before.

Reflections in Egypt

C D L LYCETT

I must admit at once that I have no clear memory of VE Day itself; certainly I recall no tremendous scenes of rejoicing, nor whatever might have been the equivalent on a Royal Air Force station in Egypt of dancing in Piccadilly Circus.

With satisfaction at the defeat of Germany there was relief that families at home would no longer be in physical danger from the war, but this was mostly unspoken and in any case the German surrender had been clearly imminent for some weeks and the V2 rocket bombardment of England had ended.

The war with Japan continued and, until it was concluded, there would be no general return home for service personnel in the middle east. Some historians of the war now believe that even if atomic bombs had not been dropped on Hiroshima and Nagasaki VJ Day would not have been much delayed, and indeed that it could have come sooner than August 1945 had the Allies not insisted upon absolutely unconditional surrender. Nevertheless, the serviceman's estimate of how long it might take was sometimes exaggerated and this modified his enthusiasm.

In the meantime the work at RAF Fayid would continue much as before VE Day, with flying training and other activities not entailing contact with enemy forces.

Turning to prevention

The RAF station at Fayid was not uncomfortable, though some little way into the desert, but it was unexciting. It overlooked the Great Bitter Lake, which was crossed by ships passing through the Suez Canal, but to which access was barred from the RAF station and the adjoining army camp. To swim, transport was needed to

97

another part of the canal, but there was a useful cricket "field" with matting wicket and a fairly firm sand outfield.

It was better to play cricket on hot afternoons than to lie under a mosquito net in the sleeping quarters. In the open air cinema the Egyptian night sky was more attractive than the films, though these were not so much bad as incongruous with the surroundings – Astaire and Rogers, with bright lights and potted palms, in the desert.

I had entered the Royal Air Force with only one house job after qualification, but with the intention of becoming a physician afterwards. It was while in the middle east that I turned to preventive medicine as a more fundamental objective. This metamorphosis was not engendered by the time honoured sanitary rounds, in which most medical officers felt professionally bound to recommend improvements clearly impossible to carry out in the circumstances; still less by the duty to ensure the daily insufflation with DDT by the sanitary squad of the more intimate recesses beneath the loose clothing of the civilian employees. An explosive outbreak of enteric fever at a dispersed site, which I was fortunate enough to control quickly, helped, but it was the conditions under which the Arab families lived in villages along the canals (used in common for defaecation, washing, and drinking) which showed how inadequate was clinical consideration of health problems by itself, in spite of the unending fascination and lower stress of clinical medicine as a career. In fairness, a reputed ten per cent pass rate in the membership examination at the end of the war, combined with the urgent need to earn a living, was a further reason.

It was this decision to enter the public health service (as it was then called) after the war which led indirectly to my meeting Dr Elston Grey-Turner for the first time – while I was county medical officer of health for Wiltshire, which was then part of his BMA territory – and to my ever increasing regard for him.

Assessment of courage

The most eventful part of the war for me had been at the beginning of my RAF service. I became the squadron medical officer to a night fighter squadron just as the Battle of Britain was approaching its climax; but I saw a good deal of the personnel of other units besides my own. We were stationed at Hornchurch and I found myself in medical charge at Rochford, which was a satellite airfield, on the famous Sunday, 15 September 1940.

About the beginning of the war the system had been introduced of psychological and psychiatric surveillance by medical officers of members of aircrews. Distinctions had to be made, for instance, between pilots who were tired or overstressed, those who had reached the point in that process when they should be temporarily rested, those who were ill, and those who merited the dire description "of low moral fibre". This duty of the medical officers, implying as it did the cultivation of a close relationship with the aircrews, must have been valuable when applied by experienced doctors who remained with stable units. With constant changes of personnel early in the war and with doctors newly qualified and commissioned, it had its difficulties. For my part, I believe that there has never been sufficient recognition of the courage and determination of aircrew generally in the Battle of Britain (many of them even less experienced in their job than I was in mine), most of the praise and publicity having gone to a few outstanding performers.

I stayed with the squadron for nearly a year after the Battle of Britain and was then posted for duties in connection with the RAF Regiment, first in medical charge at a recruit centre and then at the RAF Regiment depot where more advanced training was done. One never knew whether to take a surprise posting, accompanied by promotion or not, as a compliment to one's astonishing versatility, as a mark of displeasure, or as an operation of the ministry roulette wheel.

The makings of a regiment

The RAF Regiment was founded in 1941 to provide a ground defence force specifically for airfields. In a service where existing ground staff required technical or clerical competence, with the capacity to endure general fatigue and hardship without going sick, rather than physical fighting ability, it proved difficult for those responsible for the allocation of recruits and for setting the medical standards to comprehend the need for infantry to be fit to march, run, dig, carry weighty equipment, and to observe and shoot accurately without dependence on spectacles. They appeared to see the nascent RAF Regiment rather as a convenient destination for recruits with foot disabilities, poor eyesight, or who were unfit for service overseas (the medical grades then designated as grade II(a) (vision), grade II(a) (feet), and grade III), the "real" air force being thus relieved of them. This incongruity of medical standards for the regiment became clear during recruit training and even clearer at the RAF Regiment depot during more advanced infantry training. This led to large sick parades and general frustration of the process of forming squadrons with operational potential. We collected the medical evidence, and a battle for realistic medical standards continued for about two years as a staccato background to the routine work of running the sick quarters and dealing with sanitary matters.

The commandant of the depot was a splendid veteran who had served in each of the three armed services and apparently in a number of wars, of which he carried the facial scars. A particularly polychromatic medal ribbon among those on his tunic was rumoured to belong to the Zulu war.

He had now reappeared (a "repaint", as he was wont to say) as an air commodore. He knew all about the basic fitness requirements for infantry and took up the arguments for higher medical standards with unrelenting determination. "He used to be one of my subalterns," he would remark as he set out to tackle some remote and influential air chief marshal. At the depot he inspired much respect and affection.

Once I was summoned to the Air Ministry to put the case to the director of the RAF medical service and the assembled medical officers of the headquarters, but a more successful and lively occasion was an experiment at the depot to compare statistically the scores on the rifle range of men on grade II(a) (vision) with those of otherwise similar trainees whose visual acuity was normal. The trouble with the visually defective group, as they were quick to protest beforehand, was that, without spectacles, many of them could not see the target clearly, let alone the bull, but once convinced that disciplinary proceedings were not in prospect they cooperated with a will. Markers in the butts, with their heads well down, were left with splintered poles devoid of the marking discs, bullets ricocheted off unlikely outlying objects, and the cows in the pastures above the targets disappeared rapidly over the skyline. The result of the experiment was a statistically highly significant argument for stricter visual standards.

Eventually the right changes were made in the medical standards, and in the fit and highly efficient Royal Air Force Regiment

Huntercombe.   Tues. 1. May.
        Great public excitement as it is
known that the Germans (Himmler)
are negotiating a surrender. German
resistance has practically collapsed in
Italy (where Mussolini has been captured
by partisans and shot) and in southern
Germany. There is still a fanatical
struggle in Berlin and hard fighting
in the North near Bremen. But
the end cannot be far off.

Huntercombe.   Thurs. 3. May.
        To Worthing to-day to a demonstration
of how to issue orders to German officers.
        German power is collapsing. The
whole Army Group in northern Italy
has surrendered (over a million men)
and Parliament, Press and public are
loud in their praises and congratulations
to Alex. The Mediterranean war is
thus over. Meanwhile vast hordes
of Germans are surrendering to Monty,
Berlin has been captured, and Hitler
is dead — probably suicide. Admiral
Doenitz, rather to everyone's surprise,

From Elston Grey-Turner's diary, 1945.

is the new Führer.

There is a strange absence of
jubilation or excitement over these
tremendous news. Rather an
atmosphere of quiet satisfaction, tinged
with anxiety about the problems of
the peace.

Huntercombe.   Sat. 5. May.

All the Germans in N.W Germany,
Denmark and Holland have surrendered
to Monty. No developments in
Norway or Czecho-slovakia, and no
sign of the many pockets (Dunkirk,
St Nazaire, Channel Islands, Breslau,
Greek Islands etc) capitulating.

The Russians continue to be very
tiresome over Poland and other matters.

Denys Percy and I had a party
to-night. Drinks at Hatchett's, the
Berkeley, and the Mayfair, then a
bad dinner at Hatchetts.

Then on to collect a friend of
Denys' who took us to the Wellington
Club in Knightsbridge. Danced a

Little, then home. "Tunis Day".

Grand Hotel, Eastbourne.   Mon. 7. May.
    Came here yesterday evening to attend
a course. Very dull. There were rumours
during the day that the Germans had
finally surrendered, not confirmed. Altogether
this final surrender is so long delayed
that its arrival will be quite flat.

                "VE Day"

Grand Hotel, Eastbourne   Tues - 8. May
    To-day the official announcement
of the end of the war in Europe and
the German capitulation. A public
holiday. The Germans announced it
yesterday, and all yesterday afternoon
flags and bunting appeared on every
house. To-day we worked as usual,
but listened to the Prime Minister's
broadcast at 3 pm and to the
King at 9 and to all the
excellent commentaries by the BBC on
the crowd scenes in front of Buckingham
Palace, in Whitehall and elsewhere.
After dinner Vaughan and I walked

through this sleepy town and saw the
crowds celebrating in the pubs, and a
large crowd singing and dancing round
a bonfire on the beach.

This is a great day for Britain
and especially perhaps for Winston
Churchill, who must have received
to-day in Whitehall one of the greatest
ovations any Englishman has ever
received. He deserves it. There
appeared also to be a terrific crowd
at the Palace.

There is only one thing that mars
the day: Poland, the country for whom
we went to war nearly six years
ago, is divided and unhappy. It may
be a foretaste of difficulties to come.

of today I suppose that there is no memory of such initial obstacles.

Eventually, also, the commandant decided finally to retire and, with his departure, I was posted to the middle east. "About time, too!" was no doubt the verdict on me, and this was true.

Res Mediterraneae

A I S MACPHERSON

Dies laeta, notanda candidissimo calculo.* Such was 8 May 1945 after the sun had gone down, but during the day no hint came through to the operating room that great events were occurring. There had been heartening news of advances on the northern front as the Italian spring burgeoned, but 8 May seemed no different from any other day until the late afternoon when apparently the whole Italian population erupted on to the streets of Caserta shouting, cheering, singing, and dancing. The war in Europe was over. That Italy had played a somewhat ambivalent role in the process and was still an occupied country were not considerations likely to weigh heavily with the Italians when such a cause for celebration presented itself. In the event most of the locals reckoned it was worth about a week's holiday. By contrast our celebrations were so muted that I cannot recall any having taken place. Over a drink or two in the mess that evening what was to come next was discussed – whether we would get home, be sent to the far east or just be kept in the CMF; and speculation over what sort of a Britain awaited our return after three or four years away. Pointed suggestions I do recollect being made to the mess committee to do something to mark the occasion appropriately, which they presumably did for there appeared in the suggestion book a verse of doggerel which must be enshrined somewhere in the archives, more or less as follows:

> X – son, don't apologise
> We scarcely could believe our eyes
> We thought it was a fable.
> The mess committee, lo, has come
> Behind the tucket of your drum
> As fast as it was able.
> The suggestion you put in the book
> The mess committee and the cook
> Have laid upon the table.

*A day of rejoicing fit to be marked with the whitest of stones.

102

Speculation soon gave way to reminiscence and we fought our battles over again, remembering as is usual in times of success the pleasant and the humorous and forgetting the tribulations, frustrations, and times of utter weariness. I recalled that I had mobilised three times for this campaign – first in the delightful surroundings of Peebles hydro around mid-summer, then in a technical college in mid-Lancashire and finally in the prison at Knutsford. Our 200 bed hospital marched away through the Cheshire lanes under a full autumn moon in greatcoats, tin hats, and full kit – and three weeks later, after an extensive tour of the eastern Atlantic, marched off the ship under an African noonday sun, and in the same gear, to a sports stadium where we were to await further orders. There the steaming troops quickly discovered an open wine bar and the remainder of the day was spent "resting". Luckily the enemy had not yet spotted us and we were left alone for about 48 hours. The succeeding convoy was less fortunate and was severely mauled.

Winter 1942–3 was spent as a forward "back up" hospital for the heavy fighting in the Medjerda Valley through which the road ran almost dead straight for miles, presenting such an ideal daytime target for enemy fighters that it was called Messerschmitt Alley. Eventually in April 1943 both the First and Eighth Armies broke through, Tunis was captured, and thousands of prisoners poured back westwards packed into all manner of captured transport. The build up for the invasion of Sicily began, but circumstances allowed time first for a visit to the monastery of the White Fathers at Thibar where our hosts and guides were Brother Mungo and Brother Anthony, whose speech betrayed their origins, respectively, from the south bank of the Clyde and the south bank of the Thames; then, later, for three delightful weeks on a beach near Hammam Sousse now occupied by a large and luxurious hotel.

Forward movement

For the parachute battalion which led the way into Sicily the operation was nearly a disaster as many of them were dropped into the sea far short of their target. An old friend who was in medical charge was fortunately a strong swimmer and managed to make the shore with his heavy pack still on his back. His reply to my question why he had not jettisoned it was withering: "What, with the only bottle of whisky in it that I had seen for nine months!"

Two successive winters in Italy dispelled the myth of "sunny Italy". For part of the first we were cut off in the southern Apennines by a combination of snow and the destruction of the railway by enemy action; and in the second those who were in the north were squelching through mud almost over the top of their gumboots. Vesuvius stole the show with a major eruption in February 1944, and was still belching a plume of smoke many miles long during the day and a column of fire by night two months later when the last battle for Cassino began. The barrage which preceded the advance was deafening, but through the din came the clear and liquid notes of an Italian nightingale singing a heavenly descant to the brutish bass of the guns.

The taking of Cassino was an incredible military feat, the monastery on its very steep hill dominating and almost corking the north end of a straight and narrow valley bounded on each side by steep and barren hills. When we followed the advancing troops into the town it was in ruins, but the walls of the albergo still stood and beneath its shingle hung a notice, "Under new management". Intermittent but always forward movement took us through the centre of Italy to the southern outskirts of Perugia, where the July sun beat down so fiercely that the night operating shift was welcomed. To come out of the operating tent in the cool of the dawn and gently to climb the hill beside the camp, picking brambles on the way, was to savour one of the real pleasures of life. Another was a leisurely week spent with our transfusion officer in Florence, and a third was to return thence to find lying on my camp bed my young brother, on his way from fighting in the desert and with the Maquis to being parachuted behind the German lines to help organise the Partigiani. As an officer in the 79th he considered himself properly dressed only when he wore the kilt, which he did even when he was floating earthwards beneath a parachute.

End of an era

Shortly thereafter the increasingly glutinous mud of the Po Valley brought the fighting on the north eastern Italian front to a sticky halt and my transfer to base hospital at Caserta followed. There, long operating days interspersed with large outpatient sessions, the care of more than 100 surgical beds, and the company of specialists of all kinds made the wet winter pass quickly and it seemed no time till the whole Plain of Naples was a sheet of white cherry blossom. Then VE Day came and went and with it ended an era which none of those who survived it will forget. In the intimate sharing, over long periods, of minor triumphs and near disasters, and of boredom and enjoyment, mutual respect and tolerance were learned and friendships formed which have long outlasted the conflict, and which are kept alive by regimental reunions and by that particularly, but now no longer peculiarly, surgical institution, the travelling club.

Exciting times

REGINALD MURLEY

When I was "embodied" with my Territorial Army field ambulance in August 1939, a few days before the German invasion of Poland, I did not suspect that almost six years would pass before I could celebrate victory in Europe.

In that freezing first winter of the war I crossed France from Dunkirk to Marseilles and then, in January 1940, embarked for Haifa with some 450 horses on the SS *Talamba*, a converted British India liner. That may sound a little like setting out for the Crimea, and there was some similarity for the wives and camp followers of certain cavalry officers were not slow to join their menfolk in the Holy Land. When Italy entered the war a few months later those same ladies found that they were unable to return home, as the Mediterranean was closed to all but essential shipping.

At about that time, Elston Grey-Turner was the editor of the Barts journal and he had just published a new edition of *Round the Fountain*, an entertaining selection of its best verse contributions. I wrote to him requesting a copy of the book and he replied to say that one had been despatched. Alas, on the long and dangerous sea route around Africa, I am afraid that Elston's book never reached me.

By then the war in Europe was full of doom and gloom, but I was lucky to be serving in the more sucessful campaigns of east Africa, the middle east, and north Africa. After two years' excitement in field units I spent another two years with plastic and maxillofacial units in the Middle East and Central Mediterranean Forces. This gave rich experience to a surgeon of my tender years, and close collaboration with colleagues in neurosurgical and ophthalmic units proved of immense value to my later surgical life. These combined head and neck units were playfully dubbed "the unholy trinity" by one of our army consultants, the late Charles Donald.

After four and a half years overseas I was entitled to what was known as "python" leave. In November 1944 I returned to an England of V1 and V2 attacks, and spent three months seconded from Shenley Military Hospital to the Barts sector hospital at St Albans to brush up my general surgery.

Battle, and other, casualties

By February 1945 I was abroad again in France, working in field surgical units, firstly in Amiens and then moving with the British and American armies through Holland and over the Rhine into Germany. In mid-April I switched units to relieve a man eight years my senior who was being posted to the far east. Thus did I briefly first meet the mature, grey haired and distinguished Henry Thompson, a superb surgeon who has remained a good friend to the present day. But his team was rather disappointed by the arrival of an inexperienced and youthful looking fellow like me whom the army medical authorities, on the basis of the primary FRCS and my plastic experience, had generously made up to the status of surgical specialist. I relieved Henry at Uchte and my FSU shortly afterwards moved with a casualty clearing station to the army barracks at Lüneburg. In the few weeks before cessation of hostilities our busiest day was from midnight 29 April, when my records show that I operated upon 11 battle casualties, including three abdominal and one abdominothoracic wound.

A few days later we received British casualties from the Baltic coast. They reported that they had been shot by our gallant Russian allies. Few of us then knew that this encounter had resulted from Russian determination to occupy the Peenemünde rocket sites. On 5 May my operation book shows that I dealt with no less than seven accidental gunshot wounds. These had not occurred, as was generally the case, in battle weary soldiers keen to get out of the line, but resulted from the joyful celebrations of our troops after Admiral von Friedeburg had signed the surrender of all German forces in northwest Germany, Holland, Schleswig-Holstein, and Denmark on the previous day. Friedeburg then went on with Field Marshal Jodl to Eisenhower's headquarters at Rheims, where the final unconditional surrender became effective as from midnight on 8 May.

On the morning of VE Day we celebrated by drinking pink champagne style sparkling wine from the well stocked cellar of the German officers' mess. My only operation that day was the repair of the burst abdomen of my patient with the abdominothoracic wound whom I had dealt with nine days before. At the first operation there had been duodenal and colonic damage which had necessitated exteriorisation of the right half of the transverse colon. That burst belly on VE Day was my last battle casualty operation of the war. The patient seems to have progressed all right for I had a follow up card from one of the base hospitals on 10 June reporting, "General condition much improved. Evacuate to UK".

Such things happened

During the 10 days before we left Lüneburg news had come of the relief of Belsen concentration camp. Four of us, including the Irish colonel of our CCS, secured permission to visit the camp shortly after its liberation. Typhus was rife and we were admitted only after we had been liberally sprayed with DDT powder. The scenes in some of the huts were indescribable, with grossly emaciated occupants of both sexes and all ages, many of them suffering from dysentery and untreated injuries. The only sanitary appliances were chipped enamel bowls which were passed around the inmates practically overflowing with liquid faeces and urine. Around the huts were many more dead and dying, together with odd piles of turnips which represented the basic camp "rations". Near one end of the site were the large open pits into each of which many hundreds of pathetically emaciated corpses were crudely deposited in random and obscene disorder. The SS troops had been cleared from the neighbouring barracks to provide hospital accommodation.

Within a few days of our visit a number of British medical students were brought over to help with the feeding, nursing, and medical care of the sick inmates. Sad to say, in the early days after liberation a number of these died from overenthusiastic alimentation before the staff realised the importance of hastening slowly with their feeding.

I had my camera with me and can recall telling my companions, "I must take some pictures for my children; they will never believe that such things happened". (As a matter of fact I then had no children, and was not even remotely contemplating matrimony.)

Just before completing our tour of the camp, in stark contrast to the disturbing scenes of death and degradation, we entered a recreation hut whence we had heard the strains of music. We were astonished to find a large gathering of the fitter inmates dancing to a Hungarian band. As we left the camp, one of the Highland Light Infantry guards on the main gate asked if we would like to see his "prisoners". We inquired who they were; the guard replied, "I have Irma Grese and the doctor in here". He unlocked one cell where the notorious woman SS guard who had tortured many of the women prisoners was lying on the floor. The guard called her to attention and our colonel, overcome by his emotions, mouthed some pretty obscene expletives. We moved into the adjacent cell and there was the doctor who had despatched many of the former inmates with intravenous gasoline. Our colonel directed a further stream of rich invective at his German colleague and then spat in his face – deplorable behaviour for a British officer, one might say, but certainly understandable and excusable in those circumstances. After a further liberal spraying with DDT we returned to our unit in a dazed and unbelieving state.

A traitor spotted

Soon our CCS moved to the pleasant and undamaged city of Schleswig, close to the Danish frontier, where we had several weeks of relative quiet. With three surgical teams, and a one in three duty rota, we spent much of the time sailing yachts which our corps headquarters had commandeered from the local club. But on 21 May, three days after our arrival, there was much excitement when it was reported that William Joyce ("Lord Haw-Haw" of German propaganda fame) had been admitted. Together with several other suspects, one of whom proved to be Himmler, Joyce had been apprehended by some British troops and then suffered a through and through wound of the right buttock and penetrating wound of the left buttock when he tried to escape. He was operated upon by Buckley Hamer, and was anaesthetised by Bill Scriven, in the presence of a large audience, but, after due trial, he was hanged as a traitor on 3 January 1946. Himmler did not last so long, for he committed suicide with cyanide two days after capture.

When Joyce was admitted I had accompanied one of my colleagues to the CCS reception room, intent on hearing once more that drawling voice with which so many of us had become familiar on the German radio broadcasts. For me the experience was doubly exciting because it was one of my own original field ambulance territorials who had been among the first to spot "Haw-Haw's" identity. At the beginning of September 1939, a Sergeant Cattermole had told me that he felt sure that the man he had just heard on a German propaganda programme was an individual called William Joyce. Thereupon I sent the information to MI6. A few days later we received acknowledgement and confirmation of "Haw-Haw's" identity. Little did I then guess that I would ultimately meet this misguided traitor in Germany in such unusual circumstances.

Business as usual

JOHN NABARRO

It has to be admitted that VE Day made only a modest impact at 42 General Hospital in Haifa. The work in the outpatient clinic and caring for the multinational patients in the medical wards continued unaffected. In addition to the British we had soldiers from east African and west African pioneer corps, Arab civilians working for the army, and a few eastern European refugees who had come from Siberia through Turkey and Syria. We had two thoughts about VE Day: relief that our families in Britain would no longer be in danger from rockets – and anxiety that we might now be sent to the far east.

Although in May 1945 I was in a quiet backwater trying to get some medical experience, the earlier part of the war had been quite eventful. I qualified towards the end of 1938 and having had some training in the Officers' Training Corps while at medical school decided that I should join the Territorial Army. I was posted to 167 (City of London) Field Ambulance, which was attached to the 1st (London) Division (TA). I started my first house physician's post with Sir Thomas Lewis in February 1939 and was about to start a house surgeon's post under Mr G E O Williams when I was called up with the rest of the Territorial Army on 1 September 1939.

Defensive positions

The brigade to which we were attached was to remain in and around the City of London. Many of the soldiers in the brigade were cockneys and it was thought that if there were heavy raids on the City they would be able to help. Our task as the field ambulance was to set up a reception station where minor sick from

111

the battalions of the brigade could be looked after for a few days, all more serious cases being referred to St Bartholomew's Hospital. Our reception station was in the basement of a large building in the City and seemed reasonably equipped for its purpose. We had a steady trickle of minor infections, but the main problem was to maintain interest and morale. This phase of the war lasted two months, then the division was moved to Sussex.

The move showed up how very ill equipped we were. We had no transport of our own: the field ambulance went in charabancs with requisitioned lorries for the stores. The field artillery had some guns, but no tractors: the guns were towed to Sussex by brewers' lorries. We had good billets in the town of Uckfield. The brigade was scattered around and its prime activity was that of training. The field ambulance had a dual responsibility: training plus the establishment of a camp reception station to treat the minor sick from the brigade. We spent about three months in the Uckfield area and then moved towards Haywards Heath, where another camp reception station was set up.

This phase ended abruptly in May with the invasion of Holland and Belgium. We were suddenly provided with our own transport and moved into east Kent, the division now being expected to be in action if the Germans invaded. Shortly after this, I was seconded to divisional headquarters to understudy DADMS, Myles Formby, a distinguished ENT surgeon, who, when the authorities realised his special skills, was likely to be moved to more suitable employment. Divisional headquarters was interesting, and the head of the divisional medical services, the ADMS, was a delightful regular soldier. Work in addition to administration included sick parades for the attached units, the divisional signals, and the military police as well as divisional headquarters itself.

We had now reached the time of the Battle of Britain and Kent was the scene of many dog fights. It was also the place where German planes tended to drop their bombs if they had not managed to reach their main target, London. There were, however, very few military or civilian casualties. I was now back at the field ambulance acting as a company commander with a dressing station in Wingham, ready to handle casualties if an invasion started. This was a period of tension and as it grew more prolonged it was hard to maintain morale.

In November 1940 my company was detailed to set up a reception station for the minor sick in Canterbury and over the winter became extremely busy. We had a very large number of cases of scabies, and the nursing orderlies, mainly from the post office or clerical jobs in the City, became extremely adept at treating the condition. In February 1941 we had an epidemic of a virus infection – we called it influenza – and on one night there were as many as 135 patients in our reception station. In March I was seconded for two weeks to a casualty clearing station at Benenden girls' school. They were supposed to have a corps scabies centre and were getting very unsatisfactory results from treatment. I was instructed to take two "other ranks" and get it organised. This went quite well until I was told to hand over to the newly posted MO scabies – who turned out to be a trainee ENT surgeon.

The field ambulance moved to various locations in Kent and Sussex and then from May to November 1941 the brigade became responsible for the defence of the Romney Marsh area and Dungeness, a possible landing site for the Germans. We had a well prepared dressing station just behind the marsh, and remained prepared to handle casualties through the summer of 1941. It would appear that towards the end of that year the War Department decided that we should be withdrawn from there and prepared for overseas service. The division handed over its defensive positions and we moved to the Essex–Suffolk borders. At this time I was appointed DADMS of what had now become 56 (London) Division, with its black cat sign. Until we left England in August 1942 we had a period of intensive training, weeding out the unfit (lots of medical boards), and assembling all our equipment.

Changes of plans

Our transport and heavy stores were sent off, and then at the end of August we went by train to Liverpool. Divisional headquarters and two battalions were on one of the older prestige Cunard liners. Thirty six hours after we embarked we woke up in what those in the know recognised as the Clyde Estuary and that night we set sail in a rather slow moving but sizeable convoy with naval escort. We must have gone well out into the Atlantic, because two weeks later we woke up to find we were anchored off Freetown. No one was allowed ashore and it was hoped that keeping the ships well away from the land would obviate the risk of malaria (we were taking mepacrine). This hope was not fulfilled, and a number of cases developed two weeks later.

113

After we left Freetown, we heard about changes of plans. It had apparently been intended to send us to Egypt to reinforce the Eighth Army. Our transport and stores had been sent in a convoy to Suez. In view of the progress of the Germans on the southern Russian front, the War Department decided to divert us to "Paiforce" (Persia and Iraq Force). It would therefore be necessary to reorganise ourselves in Cape Town – our next port of call – and arrange for the transport drivers to go to Suez and the remainder of the division to Basra en route for Kirkuk in northern Iraq. The drivers would collect the transport and drive the vehicles in convoy across the Sinai and Arabian Deserts and up to Kirkuk. I was detailed to go with one field ambulance commander and the transport party – about 6000 all told – to organise the medical arrangements. The transport party embarked on the large new Dutch liner the *New Amsterdam* and made a dash for Suez unescorted. The journey was not uneventful. We sighted one submarine and relied on our speed to get away from it.

On arriving at Suez we went to transit camps near the Sweet Water Canal between Cairo and Ismailia. Then followed a hectic six weeks of getting transport and stores, visiting all the appropriate people in the medical directorate in Cairo and making the necessary medical arrangements. At the beginning of December, when most of the transport was on its way, a small group of us left independently to drive to Kirkuk. We spent three days in Palestine visiting hospitals and convalescent depots there, to try to locate divisional soldiers who had become ill in Egypt and make arrangements to get them sent back to their units. The journey from Cairo to Kirkuk is about 1400 miles and we arrived in the middle of December. Most of the road was good, but we did have trouble with rain as we approached Baghdad.

The division spent three months in Kirkuk, training vigorously in cold, unpleasant conditions. In the middle of March new orders came. We were to go in to help the Eighth Army with the First Army to finish off the Germans in north Africa. This meant a drive of some 3400 miles, which the division accomplished in 34 days.

Almost immediately on arrival we were in the front line and remained there until the Germans surrendered on 12 May 1943. Our arrival had made it possible to withdraw a division from our front and use it to outflank the Germans. We contributed in only a very small and indirect way to this victory and being a division with little experience we suffered quite heavily. We were astride the main road from Tunis to Tripoli and had to organise the movement of prisoners back. The division was then moved back to Tripoli, to re-equip and prepare for its next task, the invasion of Italy at Salerno. This was an exciting period of about three months. The last fortnight was spent in what we called "the planning house", familiarising ourselves with timetables, plans, and photographs of the beaches on which we were to go ashore.

We embarked early in September and after six days were off the shore south of Salerno. We got ashore all right and set up divisional headquarters. The medical section, at the insistence of the ADMS and with the agreement of the GOC, was always with advanced divisional headquarters – it may have been unhealthy at times, but meant that we were in close touch with operations and could deploy medical help as needed. Our progress on this landing was slow; there was much rather accurate German shelling, and a major problem was malaria; the land was marshy and mosquito control seemed to have been non-existent. We battled steadily forward on this front until we came up against the seemingly impregnable Monte Cassino and the division was rather suddenly withdrawn in February.

We thought that we should probably be pulled right out, to replace many officers and men we had lost and make good losses of stores. To our surprise, however, in the middle of February we were embarked and sent to the bridgehead established further north at Anzio. We were only there for a few weeks and we were again withdrawn. We travelled down to the south of Italy and were shipped back to Egypt, where we understood that the division was to be re-equipped and retrained before returning to Italy.

Hospital training

At this stage I had been four and three quarter years with this division. The excitement of divisional headquarters was beginning to wear thin and I was worried that I was forgetting my medicine – I had always wanted to be a physician. I talked to various people, including Neville Oswald, a physician from St Bartholomew's, who was now OC medical division at 91 General Hospital in Gaza. In June I made formal application to be transferred to a general hospital as a trainee physician. I was sent to see Evan Bedford, who was consultant physician to the Middle East Forces in Cairo, and in the middle of June I was posted to 91 General Hospital.

On arrival I was put in charge of two wards with about 40 patients. I got excellent teaching from Colonel Oswald and a locally enlisted physician, Major Ch Sheba, who was later to become head of the medical services of Israel. The patients were mainly Africans and Arabs with comparatively few from the UK. There was a wide range of clinical conditions: tuberculosis (including miliary and pericardial), malaria (especially cerebral malaria), amoebiasis, and tropical eosinophilia. Towards the end of the year we had an epidemic of infective hepatitis. I was struck by the remarkably low sedimentation rates of the patients with hepatitis (in contrast to those with malaria). I was able to show that it was due to a factor in the plasma and that the high ESR of malaria could be reduced to a subnormal level by the addition of bile salts (obtained from the pathology department) in amounts that would be expected in patients with infective hepatitis. I tried to spend part of each day in the laboratory and attended all the necropsies, of which we had quite a number. It was also possible to obtain a selection of up to date medical textbooks in Tel-Aviv and I started reading for the MRCP.

In January 1945 I was posted to 42 General Hospital in Haifa as a "graded" physician. The OC medical division there was Ronald Illingworth, the paediatrician from Sheffield. It was pleasant to be back in a city and to be able to enjoy some of the amenities of civilisation. The clinical work was again mainly with non-UK patients, but unfortunately we had a small epidemic of typhoid and a larger one of paratyphoid affecting English patients. Although VE Day came in May, most of us remained in Haifa until after VJ Day and I did not finally leave until early in December.

What had happened to mankind

LESLIE NAFTALIN

When I received a letter from the editor of the *British Medical Journal* asking me to write an article on recollections of VE Day or beforehand I was frankly stunned. The war had receded in my mind and had been replaced by many small wars since in various parts of the world, and recollections and reminiscenses only reappeared occasionally in the company of fellow officers and friends.

Six years in uniform was a long time but after nearly 40 years was a distant memory. It had been a time of excitement, fears, and foreboding, and above all, apprehension but somehow it had been removed from my thoughts by subsequent events: much has happened to me since the end of the war – restructuring my career, bringing up my family, settling down again to a happy home life with my wife after years of separation and difficulties associated with service overseas. Nevertheless, the request stimulated my thoughts and rekindled the dying embers of war memories.

Drama and confusion

The major recollection of my war service centres on the drama of the sinking of the *Bismarck* in May 1941. I was on my way to an unknown destination – a probable journey of a week or two, prolonged to seven or eight weeks by a slow convoy in the north Atlantic. As with any convoy, the ship was overcrowded, the conditions for the officers bearable, but for the other ranks poor. We gathered our information from the ship's wireless since personal radios were prohibited and when news filtered through that HMS *Hood* had been sunk, a feeling of horror passed through the whole ship. We knew that the pocket battleship could destroy our

117

whole convoy, and although we were several hundred miles away the danger was imminent. We also knew that a large part of our navy had been detailed to track and encircle the battleship, and when the final blow was struck the howl of delight that went up in the mess can never be forgotten. How can one express the feeling of relief that we all felt? We had been saved from complete destruction. The epic of the sinking of the *Bismarck* will long be a glorious chapter in the history of the British navy; it is only in retrospect that I can realise that I took part in this great drama, albeit as an onlooker. It all happened so soon after my enlistment that it was hard to believe that only a few months before I had been an assistant in general practice. What an unusual and different way of life it is to be in the army. One day you are a civilian, free to do as you wish; the next day in uniform, regimented by rules and regulations and at the mercy of your superior officer, no matter what rank you are, and so it goes on down the scale. And yet there is a companionship that develops, because in wartime everybody is in it together and if the cause is right the sacrifice is worth it.

After my initial training I realised the confusion and disorganisation of a war machine quickly mobilised. Wars are won by other nations' mistakes. I was sent to Shipton-under-Wychwood, a scenic village nestling in the Cotswolds, as the commanding officer of a motor ambulance convoy; but when I arrived I was the only member of the unit there, and I remained so for many galling weeks until one day a DADMS descended on me and asked if I had my G 1098. To his surprise I did not know what he was talking about, but eventually it came out that I should have been mobilising a unit for service overseas. It appeared that half the unit should have been with me, that is, the RAMC section, and the other half, the RASC, was mobilising in Swindon. Somehow we muddled through and within several weeks we all joined up and made our way to our port of embarkation.

During my early days in west Africa I struck up a wonderful relationship with my commanding officer. I had been transferred from the motor ambulance convoy to a field military hospital and I acted as his adjutant. We discussed at length politics, religion, sport, literature, and more mundane matters such as bridge, and this helped us to keep sane in the rather boring existence we experienced in Nigeria. Our personal contact ceased when he was posted to a unit that took part in the second front in 1943 but we maintained our friendship until he died a year or so ago at the age of 90. He was a most lovable, amiable, charming man, thoughtful and caring in times of stress, and I owe a great deal to him. I cannot believe that such friendships are possible outside the strife and torment of war conditions. I suppose these are the compensations of war.

We must never forget

I find it difficult after so many years to recollect any particular action or personal feelings on VE Day itself. I was not taking part in any active army service at the time and was a duty MO in an army base in Scotland, mainly occupied in the demobilisation of army camps and reception stations. As the destruction of the German army continued the day of my own demobilisation drew nearer. Far away and above my personal feeling, however, there was the overwhelming relief that Hitlerism was being crushed and that evil despotic rule was being annihilated for a "thousand years". My mind recalled the tragedy of the holocaust with the destruction of six million Jews, known to all thinking, liberal minded people but the full extent of the tragedy not yet being fully realised. Even now after 40 years the whole story of the brutality, the decimation of European Jewry, and the long lasting effect on the victims, has not yet been fully documented. I cannot believe that it will ever be, although archives have been founded in many countries in the world, especially Israel and the United States. We must never forget this tragedy and it must be remembered every year by the Jewish people all over the world just as they have recited the redemption from Egypt yearly at Passover for the last 2500 years.

I am sure the humanity which was part of Elston Grey-Turner would appreciate these thoughts.

So what are the real recollections of VE Day? Not one of personal things, but more of what had happened to mankind. In my lifespan I had lived through two world wars, innumerable small conflicts, and many revolutions in dozens of countries. The struggle for a better standard of living was on the move and in Britain publication of the Beveridge Report gave great hope for so many people for the future. Included was the plan for a national health service. The welfare state changed people's attitudes and although, because of economic problems, inroads have been made in the scheme, it stands out throughout the world as a beacon of hope for the future of mankind. Also the turmoil caused throughout Africa and Asia at this time gave rise to nationalism and independence for these emergent states and the possibility of a state for the Jewish people. These were the thoughts that flowed through my mind on VE Day. Forty years on have we advanced in justice, humanity, and freedom in the brotherhood of man as we would have wished? I wonder.

Among the tall trees

RICHARD NELSON

On VE Day I found myself in a stand of very tall trees in the Canadian Rockies. This may seem to be an unusual place for an RAF officer while there was a war on, but it is easily explained.

In 1943 I had been posted to the United Kingdom Air Liaison Mission, Ottawa, to act as medical liaison officer to the staff of DMS, RCAF, and also to report back on research work or other developments which might be of interest to the RAF.

In the course of this second activity I became interested in a small parachute unit stationed in Alberta. Four members of this unit were making the then incredible claim that they could control the course of their chutes and could land within feet of a target on the ground. I had visited them in the early spring and seen them make guided landings as claimed. The possibilities of the technique in reaching a crashed aircraft in difficult terrain were obvious.

They did not use the standard RAF parachute with quick release harness. Their harness had four steel rings on the central portion instead of the quick release box; it was secured by four snap hooks, each of which was fastened to its appropriate ring. The canopy looked most unsafe as there was a gap where one of the panels should have been. The shroud lines were arranged in four groups, each ending in a steel ring. The parachutist's harness had four straps leading upward, each ending in a snap hook – when these were fastened to the rings of the shroud lines all was ready for use.

After my first visit they let me know that they could land in trees and descend safely to the ground. By this time I had been posted to Washington, but in view of much of the terrain over which the RAF was operating in the far east this was obviously important and explains why I found myself in a stand of the tallest trees that could

121

be found in that part of the Rockies.

I think it was while we were waiting for the aircraft to drop its parachutists that the news of the German surrender was relayed to us, but this was of secondary importance just then.

In due course our four parachutists landed in the treetops and were suspended well over 100 feet above the ground. Each man had a coil of about 300 feet of light, strong rope attached to his belt. He proceeded to thread one end of this through the four rings of his harness fastening, being careful not to undo any of the snap hooks which held him in the harness. He then carried the same end of the rope up to the rings attached to the parachute shrouds, passing it through three and tying it securely to the fourth, and dropped the other end of the rope – being very interested to see that it reached the ground. He was then able to release himself from the canopy by undoing the snap hooks attached to the shroud rings. This left him suspended only by the rope, but the friction of its passing through the four rings of his harness ensured that he reached the ground safely at a sedate pace.

Once we were sure that our four men were safe and unhurt we were able to give our minds to the major news of the day.

With the Gunners

DONALD OLLIFF

> War lays a burden on the reeling state,
> And peace does nothing to relieve the weight.

Cowper may have been right, but peace in Europe in 1945 certainly came as a relief to most of the soldiers, and especially to those of us who were doctors.

After the grievous losses at Arnhem the 1st Airborne Division had been rebuilding its strength, and training for another landing in Europe. We who had had the good fortune to escape from Holland in 1944 felt a great obligation to get back to the war. The continuing advance of our invasion armies made this seem increasingly unlikely, however.

VE Day found us briefed for that most happy task, the liberation of Norway and Denmark. I was medical officer to the 1st Air Landing Light Regiment Royal Artillery, an exciting and satisfying life. We were stationed at Boston in Lincolnshire but training took us all over the country from the Wash to Wales, from Suffolk to Scotland. The regiment fired 24 little guns of 3 in calibre and the round weighed about 13½ lbs. They could drop them into a bucket at 6000 yards. The guns were drawn by those lovable wartime vehicles, the jeeps. Gun, jeep, and trailer were loaded into a Horsa glider. My regimental aid post had a glider loaded with a jeep and trailers with stretcher attachments. The Horsas looked to me like giant elephant hawkmoth caterpillars with great fierce faces and black swollen bodies. We were towed by Stirling or other bombing planes. The noise in flight was tremendous, but when the great lever in front was pulled to disconnect the tow rope the glider seemed to soar up and up, in utter silence and peace. I found the landings more exciting than parachuting. Suddenly the nose went down in a very steep dive, and the jeep and trailers seemed to be hanging on the little side chains with which we fixed them to strong points in the fuselage. The landscape rushed up to meet us. Then there was a great roaring hiss of escaping air as huge flaps came down to check the dive. Tree tops rushed past at 100 miles an hour. Then with a great bump we landed and raced across the fields at 70 miles an hour, crashing through hedges as though they were tissue paper.

BMJ in the mess

Looking back after nearly 40 years, most of them spent in country practice, I marvel that life then seemed so busy. All my patients were fit men. Probably more than half the day was spent in soldiering duties rather than the practice of medicine. Sick parades were small. Ten men, perhaps, were seen before breakfast. Few serious conditions turned up, and psychological problems were unusual. Officers and men were all volunteers. During the day I visited a few men, sick in their billets, lying on the floorboards in their camouflaged sleeping bags. I also visited the local hospitals, and there were always accidents. The few serious cases were admitted to the EMS hospital in Lincoln. When a fit young battery captain coughed up blood and purulent sputum upon the snow, during field firing in the Cheviot Hills, we took him back to Boston; penicillin was obtained from Sheffield University. I think it was a calcium salt, red, and injected every three hours. He did well, but in retrospect I think this was a virus pneumonia.

I had a copy of the Beveridge Report in those days, and read it eagerly. It read like one of the Old Testament prophets. I still read them with pleasure, but Beveridge has not stood the test of time. The prediction that demand falls with assiduous treatment has been proved wrong by the National Health Service – 1948 is a sad year in my book. I also read the *BMJ* eagerly, and scanned longingly the advertisements for hospital jobs which were not for me; I used to leave it in the mess as a talisman, just as others left their sporting journals, literary reviews, or glossy social magazines.

Life in the mess was happy. We ate and drank like kings; probably the great amount of exercise we took prevented us from getting fat. The mess sergeant was sent to London regularly to buy delightful foods which were not rationed; we also shot wild fowl on the fens. The talk was good. The officers came from widely differing backgrounds but the atmosphere was brotherly and relaxed; Christian names were used freely. In addition to a VC, there were many DSOs and MCs. One of the subalterns had a ribbon for helping to carry the King's train at the coronation. I wrote to my father, "The padre and I feel rather naked about the chest, with only our NAAFI and campaign gongs up".

Boston cheer

Over this vigorous scene soared the enormous tower of St Botolph's Church. One freezing day a small party of us climbed up into the great lantern, more than 250 feet above the market place. The stone was icy and the wind screamed in from the fens and the sea. But there was nothing cold in the relationship between the Gunners and the town. I have often wondered how many marriages took place after the war. I remember the friendship and hospitality of the local doctors. They were working harder than I was, but they found time to welcome a junior colleague in uniform. One evening just before VE Day the regiment was returning from an exercise. The jeeps were all open, without hoods or windscreens, to save weight in the air. They were crammed with troops. There was a fair in the market place, and a considerable crowd. As the convoy wound its way through, our little pennants fluttering on the wireless aerials, and the late sun gilding the Boston Stump, someone started to cheer. The people cheered the troops and the troops cheered back. Cheer upon cheer, the whole town rang with this happy sound. Soldier and civilian alike, we all knew the end of the war in Europe was very near, and longed for the brave new world to come. One day I must go back to Boston – the echoes of those cheers can have never quite died away.

Very soon after this about 6000 airborne troops flew to Norway to round up 350 000 German troops. The first atomic explosion had not taken place, and many of us were thinking of the battles to come in the far east – especially the retaking of Singapore. We left our little guns behind in England. I wonder if they ever fired again? The total fire power of that gallant regiment, with all its guns, jeeps, gliders, and hundreds of men must have been much less than that of one modern missile.

*   *   *

I cannot end this slight contribution without mentioning Elston Grey-Turner. He was there at the BMA when I used to go up as local medical committee representative. He was always the same, whether at the BMA or the Apothecaries' Hall: gentle and unruffled, a distinguished figure in any company. I don't know if it's true that the real strength of the BMA lies in its backwoodsmen. True or not, he knew our names, and made us welcome in the stately precincts of London. I saw him last at the Toronto meeting in 1983. By chance we sat together at the Christian breakfast to hear a memorable talk. Soldier, administrator, and diplomat, but always the physician; we shall not see his like again.

A mixture of feelings

A E PORRITT

It was a bright, sunny crisp morning in Brussels – so I walked from the Twenty first Army Group headquarters mess in the beautiful tree lined Avenue Louise (a block of luxury flats that we had taken over from the SS when we arrived before Christmas 1944, but from which we had never quite succeeded in eradicating that peculiar individualistic smell that seemed to permeate through all buildings occupied by German military units) to headquarters in the massive Shell building overlooking the famous Grand Place in the centre of the city, where, as consulting surgeon to Twenty first Army Group, I had a somewhat spartan office on the fourth floor (I think it was). Its bareness was due to the fact that I only occupied it for brief periods of a day or two (to keep up with the everlasting paperwork that even in the midst of an active war never seems to cease proliferating), between protracted trips to visit forward surgical units in the battle zone and the many hospitals and allied institutions in the ever expanding "lines of communication" areas.

Almost an anticlimax

It was also 8 May 1945 – VE Day. We had heard rumours of the impending collapse of the German forces for some days, but it was not until mid-morning on that day that a rapidly increasing deep rumble of noise from the square penetrated even the double glazed windows of my office – to be followed very soon by an excited messenger bearing the official news of complete surrender. Quite honestly, it produced in me, alone in my quiet office, a weird mixture of feelings: obviously relief and rejoicing, as was so evident in those milling crowds below, combined with an odd sense of regret that this magnificent effort was now over (officially) and that this superb, challenging, exciting job of mine was now to

127

be wound up. The stimulating tension of the past 12 months suddenly went flat; there was a sense almost of anticlimax.

But I had to do something. Having noisily visited those of my colleagues in other branches who were in the building, I ordered my car and drove out through a city gone mad to one of our larger hospitals near Brussels – 113 General at Lisieux – where one of my greatest personal friends, Lieutenant Colonel William Copeman (the "father of rheumatology" in Britain) was in charge of the medical division. We duly lunched and celebrated with champagne in his mess – but somehow I sensed that negative "end of term" feeling had crept in here too. So I went on with my faithful Welsh driver, Jones (who had been with me since Normandy and was ultimately to drive me home when I was demobilised from our then German headquarters in Bad Herford to my flat in Regent's Park), to a small field hospital, 96 General, at nearby Tournai to which I had become very attached since they had housed me temporarily on the Normandy beachhead. There we continued to celebrate – together with patients who were "feeling no pain at all" – and listened to Churchill's speech.

The evening I spent with some Belgian friends at their home – our quietly happy celebratory dinner being augmented by some special NAAFI "rations" I had been able to obtain, and some excellent Traminer wine that had been carefully hidden and treasured over the years in preparation for such an occasion. I had met this charming and hospitable family when I first arrived in Brussels, chasing hotfoot my forward surgical units that had "leapfrogged" their way behind the British and Allied tank force on its headlong drive from the Normandy beachhead, through France to Belgium.

In December 1944, during that very dangerous last German thrust into the Ardennes, whilst visiting units in that wooded, snow covered, difficult scene of action, I had been able to "rescue" the six year old son of my friends from his grandmother's isolated chateau where he had been sent for his Christmas holidays. I do not imagine that young lad will ever forget his perilous long drive on wintry roads – sitting proudly beside Jones – back to Brussels, and being delivered to his much relieved mother about 2.30 am. After that their home was a home from home for me during my many transient visits to Brussels, and perhaps it was fitting that I should spend my VE night of somewhat mixed feelings in that friendly family atmosphere.

Activity and excitement

I think my rather negative reaction was enhanced by the fact that the previous five or six weeks had been a period of intense activity, of great interest, and of much excitement. They had included the Rhine crossing – so long awaited; the first harum scarum journey into Germany, a sadly devastated and dreary Germany with its sullen, dull eyed frightened people; a visit – forever imprinted on my soul – to the horror of the Belsen concentration camp in the first few days after its "relief"; a comprehensive tour of Belgian and Dutch units to arrange transference to Germany; a couple of days in Paris at a surgical conference with the Americans, and my opposite number, Colonel Elliott Cutler; a quick dash over to London to report to the War Office and put in a brief appearance at the Association of Surgeons meeting. Little wonder, therefore, that there was a sense of anticlimax, an "it's all over" feeling. I was soon on the road again, however, the next day visiting units in Belgium, Holland, and – even more extensively – Germany.

To add a little more excitement to the scene, I had to deal with the commander in chief who had sustained a minor back injury when his light plane had "pancaked" while paying a visit to Canadian troops in Denmark. Field Marshal Montgomery was a highly inquisitive patient, but, once cognisant of the position, an equally docile and cooperative one – as I had reason to appreciate on two or three other postwar occasions when I was privileged to help him with minor surgical problems.

The problems of demobilisation soon became obvious. I conducted Lord Moran on a comprehensive tour of Twenty first Army Group medical units, whilst he tried to explain to rather dubious medical officers what a civilian future held in store for them. My own demobilisation was delayed from June, when it was officially due, to October as the post of consulting surgeon was classified as a "key post" to which normal demobilisation procedures would not apply. This did, however, give me the fascinating experience of observing at first hand the transition in a conquered country from military to civilian administrations.

My last leisurely, protracted, nostalgic tour of what for 15 exciting months had been my "parish" (down to the Normandy beaches, back through France, Belgium and Holland, and Denmark to Berlin, and finally to our headquarters near Lüneburg in Germany) underlined for me what a unique and magnificent experience this had been. The superlative work, the loyalty and happy friendships of my large surgical team, the understanding and ready help of the regular RAMC, the efficiency and cooperation of the other branches of the Army Group – and of their leaders, from the C in C downwards, made it all an unforgettable saga. Yes, in perspective, VE Day was a very special day – a wonderful day.

Scenes of action

FRANK RICHARDSON

Memories of VE Day? I suppose these would be most vivid among those who had been "abed in England" – all that mafficking, splashing about in Trafalgar Square, and so on. For those of us lucky enough to have been where it was all happening the great day itself tends to be obscured by other memories. But no army doctor with affectionate memories of that great and wise man would willingly opt out of a tribute to Elston Grey-Turner. So I'll settle for a few experiences around VE Day.

The end in sight

I was ADMS of 15 (Scottish) Division, which had played centre-forward in the advance into and through Germany – the Reichs-wald and the Siegfried Line, assault crossings of the Rhine and Elbe. That last battle had been a tough one, with kamikaze like pilots flying last ditch sorties from the Hamburg autobahn, but we felt sure that the end was in sight. Soon after our successful crossing the first overture of surrender was made to our division, and our divisional commander, Colin Barber – six feet eight or nine inches, and inevitably nicknamed "Tiny" – conducted the Chief of Staff of Army Group Blumentritt to the headquarters of 8 Corps, as the second step in a process which was to escalate to Lüneburg Heath, and the well publicised surrender ceremony. Our general was determined to have absolutely no publicity at our end. So when the CRA, Brigadier Lyndon Bolton, and I decided that we could not bear to miss so historic a scene, we kept well out of the way, hiding in bushes and even swapping headgear in case the general should spot us (Brigadier Bolton was the only officer in the division who did not wear a Balmoral bonnet). Prep school stuff perhaps but a "last day of term" spirit was in the air.

Brigadier Harry Cumming-Bruce (later Major General the Lord Thurlow) a Seaforth Highlander with a fine flair for leadership, had published his operation order for the Elbe crossing in three colours, Allied flags and all, and defined his intention to lead the division across the Elbe and advance to the Baltic, there to provide "a firm base for postwar planning". I had come across Harry Cumming-Bruce in Goch, the first town in Germany which we overran, whilst he was replenishing his supply of towels in a looted draper's shop. "Well, Frank," he said, "what can you expect from a descendant of the man who looted the Elgin Marbles?" I did not then know enough about that alleged rape to be able to tell Harry that his great forebear had saved the marbles from Turkish neglect and paid for them out of his own pocket. In Goch I saw a nice example of our public relations campaign. Among the mounds of impassable rubble to which most of the unlucky town had been reduced, was a poster prophesying, in German and English: " 'Give me five years and you will not recognise Germany' – Adolf Hitler."

Soon after the end of hostilities was announced we members of the general's mess were sitting at breakfast in a small house in the hamlet of Hammoor, a few miles from Ahrensburg, where we eventually established our headquarters in the schloss. To our amazement a column of SS armoured vehicles drove slowly down the main – well, the only – street. The soldiers appeared to be well disciplined; their weapons bristled a few feet from our table. Neither we nor, so far as I can remember, the divisional defence platoon did a damned thing about it. We later learned that this formation, refusing to accept their nation's surrender, had "holed up" in the Forest of Segeberg, through which I was soon to drive, on my way to sort out the medical problems in the great port of Kiel, occupied by our 46 Brigade. I was advised to drive through the forest as fast as I could without stopping, but, as usual, found it irresistible to get out and question the wandering tribes who swarmed everywhere in those troubled days – displaced persons of many lands, and parties of Germans, who had obviously been soldiers, all with one urgent impulse: to get as far away as they could from the Russians.

In Kiel I found that, in contrast to the disintegrating discipline of the German army, their navy preserved some self respect and good order. Incidentally, once across the Elbe the stiffest resis-

tance which we had encountered had been from young marine
cadets from Hamburg, many of them still mere boys. I needed to
give only two orders to the German surgeon admiral: his sailors
were to shave daily unless they had his permission to "grow" (I
thought this sounded commendably "naval"); and, secondly, to
put a stop to nightly carousing, especially among his officers, all
alcohol, apart from a suitable allotment for "hospital comforts",
was to be handed over to me. I expected a few cases to put into the
boot of my car and was just a little set aback when he asked when
the transport would be available. In the end I settled for a lorry
load of assorted bottles, with which I made a fairy godmother
round of our units. I later regretted that I had not "acquired" (the
term "liberated" was also popular) a fine pair of Zeiss binoculars. I
had taken only a couple of officers' dirks – one for each, as yet
unborn, son.

In defeat

On the Sunday after VE Day passers by would have heard a
mighty male voice chorus swelling from the church of Ahrensburg,
as we sang "Now thank we all our God". If this purloining of the
Germans' own great hymn of thanksgiving "Nun danket Alle
Gott" (Johannes Crüger: 1598–1662) rubbed salt into the wounds
it was, I am sure, unintentional – unlike that poster in Goch. If any
passing German thought wistfully of the days when Frederick's
Prussians made their victorious battlefields ring with that wonderful sound, German soldiers singing, I doubt if many inside the
church spared a thought for the days when our soldiers must have
heard it sung by their German allies, as at Minden and Waterloo.

Such thoughts were banished from our minds, temporarily at
least, by the pathetic indeed almost awe inspiring, spectacle of that
great army in total defeat, streaming westward, leaving every field
in which they had slept littered with straw and hay, of which the
farmers would bitterly resent the loss in the coming months. The
stern antifraternisation edict stifled any expression of sympathy;
and indeed any stirring of comradeship towards the beaten enemy
(such as would have been possible in our old western desert days
with the soldierly men of the Afrika Korps) had died under the
impact of Belsen and similar atrocities. I consider myself lucky not
to have had to enter Belsen in those early days; the experiences of

those who did so make horrific reading.* The Germans had begun an attempt to conceal the magnitude of this crime, and a train load of the victims had been dumped in a hutted camp near Celle when the train taking them deeper into Germany was bombed. A Gunner colonel was close to tears when he told me about the situation demanding my attention. The all too familiar pictures of Belsen spare me the need to attempt a description of what I then saw – living skeletons lying among dead ones, a scene of almost literally indescribable horror.

The impact of that spectacle enables me to justify to myself the harshness with which I treated the inhabitants of Celle and the two senior German army doctors, whom we compelled to do what was necessary under our supervision. The citizens had to fill the lorries, which I sent round, with their best clothing and bedding, and food for the robuster ex-captives (the most serious cases needed special diets). The German officers (of equivalent ranks to brigadier and lieutenant colonel) themselves carried out the corpses for burial. When I had to depart and hurry after our advancing division the senior medical officer begged me with tears in his eyes, "as a doctor" to believe that he had known nothing of this dreadful camp. He had, after all, thousands of German soldiers as patients in the hospitals under his control. I told him that I did believe him, and asked him, as a doctor, to do all he could for the survivors of his compatriots' brutality and neglect.

European spirit

That German plea, "We didn't know", was to become increasingly familiar in the post Nazi era; but I felt growing satisfaction that I had accepted that German doctor's word when, during the early postwar years, I saw how unsatisfactory conditions could insidiously creep in even under our supposedly civilised administration. Writing about all this in 1975, in *Blackwood's Magazine*, I called the article "Natural allies", for that was the term which Sir Archibald Allison had used for the Germans in that magazine in 1836. If it was possible to use that term in 1975 it certainly was not in 1959, when our plans to celebrate, with the Germans, the 200th anniversary of the Battle of Minden were stamped upon very firmly by General de Gaulle.

*See *J R Army Med Corps* 1984; **130**: 34–59.

Now, surely, what with the EEC and all that, our country which, during centuries of changing alliances, has fought both by the side of and against most of the members of the Community, should be able to play a useful role in fostering a European spirit and what I like to call, on the military side, esprit de Nato.

Home service

J S RICHARDSON

My wife and I were on leave in Cornwall on VE Day. We were staying in a small private hotel, the owner of which had great pride in his ancient tin mine. At his insistence we visited it with him, the entrance surrounded by gorse blazing in the sunshine with silence all around us. On our return to the hotel we heard of the end of the war in Europe.

It was strangely unreal. For six years we had longed for this moment, and now it had come and we happened to be in a place seemingly remote both in time and space from the urgency of war – sun, silence, and the old tin mine.

Our children, aged eight and five, were with their nanny in Aldershot and they saw real military celebrations under her strict but loving supervision. What really impressed them was that they had "a flag each", not just one to share as had been their lot in most things in the latter years of the war.

Medical experience

They were in Aldershot because I had been posted as officer in charge of the medical division at the Cambridge Military Hospital at the end of October in the previous year. I was naturally much disgusted at being graded category C (home service only) by a medical board after being invalided from north Africa on a stretcher. But in the event the posting was a marvellous medical experience before returning to civilian practice. It taught me things that were to be important to me in my later years about administration by clinicians and the results that could be got in cost effective terms for patients from the thoughtful use of scarce resources.

The top administration of the Cambridge was of high quality and there was no interference in clinical matters. The commanding officer was a retired colonel, Mickey O'Readon, a small dapper bachelor with an Irish brogue and happy memories of service in India in times of peace when "There was plenty of horses, a little soldiering, and no bloody doctoring". He had two special advantages for an officer in charge of a division. He disliked the local assistant director of medical services, who had served under him in the prewar days; and he always exploded in fury if it was suggested that an army hospital did not rate with a civilian one. These admirable qualities could be used to advantage in getting initially opposed construction work carried out or equipment purchased.

The matron was a small, amusing, somewhat acid regular QA who terrified the girls but had a proper preference for the men. Miss Alban's Christian name, Henrietta, somehow suited her, and my wife and I were happy that we could keep up to some extent with her and with the colonel until they died.

The building was a pleasant one in which to work, with light, airy, Nightingale type wards and wide corridors. The officer patients' block was modern and the outpatient facilities adequate for several specialists to work in at the same time.

VIPs and prisoners

Because of the effects of the bombing of London and especially the recent unmanned flying bomb (doodlebug) assaults, the Cambridge Hospital was at that time the main reference hospital at home for both VIP officers and special medical or administrative problems.

Among these were two large wards full of Russians who had been prisoners of war under the Germans and had been released by the Allies as they crossed Europe. This was medically alarming as many had open pulmonary tuberculosis and were in urgent need of treatment. All were really ill. It was surprising to find the effect in raising morale of the mere sight of an artificial pneumothorax apparatus and the showing of an active interest in them. The story had, however, an unfortunate ending for me as I became infected, and an appalling one for the patients: they had to be handed over to the Russians on instructions from on high.

They knew what this meant and we, less informed, became nevertheless fearful for them on the arrival of Russian medical officers, the grandeur of whose uniforms was only matched by their total lack of interest in their men and their medical circumstances. It sickened us, as the poor men really thought we could have helped them.

An unusual minor medical problem was presented by another group of prisoners, this time Germans. They had been brought over from the Channel Islands, where they had been in the occupying force. Great was our surprise when we saw that a number of them had a remarkably intense yellow discoloration of their palms. It was quite unlike mepacrine discoloration of the skin or any other rare condition such as chronic arsenical poisoning. Carotenaemia seemed the only explanation and proved to be the case.

Their story was that they had become convinced they had no hope of being relieved from the islands before Germany was defeated, and were conscious of the hatred that surrounded them. They decided that urgent self interest demanded the creation of some good will so they handed over their rations to the local population and repaired to the fields to forage for root vegetables and anything else they could find to keep them alive. They were a miserable, half starved, elderly lot who were moved on shortly to a POW camp, and unfortunately we lost sight of their response to replacement therapy.

Russians and Germans were not the only prisoners who gave us interest and work. The inmates of the local military prison, the "glasshouse", kept the prisoners' ward full and gave experience in malingering on a scale beyond that of the single individual. There was, for instance, an epidemic of methaemoglobinaemia that provided a dramatic clinical picture for the inexperienced. It was due to ingesting anti-gas ointment. This nuisance was brought to an end when a dramatic midnight refusal to allow a man to be treated was only reversed after the sergeant major, with great histrionic skill, pleaded for the man's life and convinced the horrified occupants of the prisoners' ward of the mortal danger that further cases would run. The ceremonial intravenous injection of methylene blue added conviction to the act.

It was from this kind of local problem, from the struggles of unit commanders to coerce the doctors into letting them return to their commands while still unfit, as well as from an endless volume of more routine medical work, boards, and clinical problems that I was relaxing on VE Day in blissful peace and idleness.

138

Postgraduate rehabilitation

The reality of actual peace was, of course, an anticlimax. Nevertheless there was an increasing interest as the Cambridge became a kind of postgraduate medical rehabilitation centre. In addition to the staff on the establishment, some of whom were anxious to sit the examination for MRCP, there were lieutenant colonels, majors, and graded specialists posted to the division who had been either prisoners of war or off sick for prolonged periods. In addition there was a brigadier who had been in Burma and wished to get back into clinical work after distinguished active service.

They were a remarkable group, and at least three became the holders of major consultant appointments in the National Health Service. Such quality raised the standards of clinical care to a high level and it was not surprising that they compared not unfavourably with those we found on returning to our civilian hospitals. This is a proud boast but I think Colonel Elston Grey-Turner would have criticised us and laughed at us but have thought the unit was a good one.

Of things (partly) remembered

HENRY ROLLIN

There could have been no more appropriate setting for the drama enacted on Sunday 3 September 1939 than the events that immediately preceded it. That night there was an electric storm the like of which I have never seen before or since. Lightning, which seemed to be sustained indefinitely, turned night into day. What, strangely enough, heightened the awesome show of pyrotechnics was the virtual lack of thunder and rain.

At that time I was a junior member of the staff of a mental hospital in Surrey, a hospital given over to the care of what were then known as "mental defectives". The hospital was gloriously located high on the Downs and surrounded by undulating woodlands and farmland. Strategically it was less blessed: its grounds were separated by a low fence from the Guards' depot, and a mere 1000 yards as the Messerschmitt flew from RAF Kenley, one of a number of fighter stations designed to defend London from the Luftwaffe.

On the morning of 3 September, quite spontaneously, the entire medical staff, resident and non-resident, forgathered in the mess to hear the official declaration. Stuart Hibberd, the doyen of BBC radio newscasters (then known as "wireless announcers"), with his mellifluous voice and perfect diction, introduced the Prime Minister. At 11.15 Chamberlain sounding, understandably perhaps, more lugubrious than ever, declared that because Germany had not replied to England's ultimatum (and who in their right senses ever thought she would?) the two countries were at war. There followed an awkward silence which was broken by the banshee wail of the air raid siren. The war was on.

Baptism of fire

The "phoney" war, the sitzkrieg, was followed by the blitzkrieg, and our baptism of fire. Because of the hospital's location we came in for far more than our fair share of the action. Both the Guards' depot and Kenley were legitimate targets, but any slight inaccuracy in the bombing, for whatever reason, meant that we were one of the likely recipients of the straying missiles. There was a minor compensation, however: from our vantage point we could watch in daylight the dog fights between the fighter planes of the RAF and the Luftwaffe. Tin hats were mandatory to protect our skulls from the spent cartridges that hailed down from the cloudless skies.

Because of the deteriorating military situation the appropriate BMA committee was obliged to change its policy and allow doctors in hospitals in and around London, hitherto "frozen", to join the forces. I was the first in my hospital to be "unfrozen". I was commissioned in the RAF in June 1941. Before leaving I did a round of my wards. From the male nurses, many of them ex-Guardsmen, I collected handshakes and some good advice, given with many a nudge and a wink. From the ward sisters, some of them tear stained, I collected an extraordinary assortment of gifts, including bars of chocolate, and, hand knitted with loving care, a pair of mittens, a balaclava helmet, two pullovers, and several pairs of thick wollen socks, concealed in one of which was a ten shilling note.

It may sound sacrilegious, but having transmuted my scalpel into a sword, I enjoyed my war. It was an honour – I use that word advisedly – to belong to an elite corps, the courage and skill of whose airmen I had witnessed at first hand with drooling admiration.

My first posting was to a flying training school in the very heart of the Cotswolds, thus beginning a continuing and ever deepening love affair with that most gentle, beguiling, and seductively beautiful garden in all England. In addition to its unique setting, RAF Rissington was my first, and indeed, my only experience of a peacetime mess. There could be few five star hotels that could compare with it. But for me, it was the deep, deep peace pervading the place that grabbed me, a dramatic change from the wailing sirens, the bombs, the high level of anxiety, and the disturbed nights that, as a civilian, I had left behind.

End of an idyll

This idyll ended after six months in circumstances that served to prove that, even if you are right, it doesn't pay to argue with regular group captains, even medical ones. I was posted within 24 hours, and in the bitter winter of 1941–2 I was downgraded to the status of an itinerant locum, filling in for a week here, a week there at various stations while the regular MO was sick or on leave. More often than not I had to live in billets and, as I was to learn, the range of billets was enormous. I can remember, for example, a baronial mansion where I dined off a somewhat meagre portion of Welsh rarebit elegantly served by a liveried butler; and a two up two down terrace house where the pinafored housewife served a sumptuous three course "high tea".

Psychiatry, as a discipline distinct from, or complementary to, neurology, came to be recognised in the RAF in the early 1940s. It came to light that I had had some psychiatric experience and held the DPM. I was rescued from my servitude and deemed a "neuropsychiatrist". Thereafter I applied myself as best I could to the various jobs I was called upon to do, both routine and research. The last three years of my service, however, were spent at the Central Medical Establishment, Cleveland Street, W1, located immediately opposite the Middlesex Hospital.

There was no mess and I was required to find my own accommodation. This presented no problem. In those days highly desirable furnished accommodation was on offer at ludicrously low rentals. I shared a bijou mews house near Regent's Park with a brother officer employed at the same establishment. But living in London, in effect as a civilian, and working office hours, meant that the close identification with the RAF ceased. It was, therefore, in this hybrid state that I shared with other Londoners the fluctuating fortunes of war during those fateful years, 1944 and 1945.

Few would doubt that D Day, 6 June 1944, was the most critical day of the war. What was so remarkable was that the preparations for this, the most ambitious and complex military operation ever mounted, were kept so secret. Certainly I, walking the corridors of power (or so I thought), had not the slightest inkling of what was going on. On the day of the initial landings on the Normandy coast, and subsequent days, we lived with our ears glued to the wireless in a state of suspended animation. It was a triumph; and in less than a year, the impregnable fortress that Germany thought she had built on the continent of Europe crumbled. Victory in Europe

142

was not so much a matter of if, but when.

VE Day, when it came, was something of an anticlimax. All day on Monday 7 May 1945, we waited for the official announcement. But there was muddle and delay. Perhaps there was trouble in the celestial stage management department. Surely, anything so momentous as the declaration of peace deserved the same special effects as the declaration of war. And so eventually it came to pass: on the night of 7/8 May there was another electric storm, this time, however, accompanied by more thunder and torrential rain than its predecessor.

Emotional lid off

Tuesday 8 May was to be the day. Winston Churchill was to broadcast at 3 pm and the King at 9 pm. Dutifully I and my flatmate turned up at Kelvin House; but work was unthinkable. About lunchtime we decided to go AWOL. Living and working in the west end for three years meant that we had come to know, and to be known, in a variety of restaurants and pubs in the locality. We had no definite plan but decided to make our way in the direction of Buckingham Palace which, in the nature of things, was bound to be the focal point of the celebrations. We ambled down Charlotte Street, across Oxford Street, downing the odd one or two en route in one or two haunts; then the automatic pilot took over and we found ourselves in our favourite lunchtime pub just off Shaftesbury Avenue. Crowds were beginning to gather, but movement was possible.

Eventually – how much later I have no idea – we emerged into bright sunshine, turned into Shaftesbury Avenue, and headed west into Piccadilly and beyond. It was the atmosphere that I recall best. The emotional lid was off: London with total abandon had let down her hair, lifted her bedraggled skirts, and danced a fandango – quite literally where space permitted.

As we progressed – a soft shoe shuffle is a more appropriate description – the crowds grew thicker, but we eventually made it, and even found room on the steps of the Victoria Memorial (I could identify myself in a picture published in the press the following morning).

The scene was unbelievable and indescribable, but not, unfortunately, unforgettable. I say not unforgettable because, truth to tell, I have forgotten a good deal: and for this impairment of memory I blame the demon drink with a splash of Anno Domini. There are islets of memory, however, although I would not guarantee the chronological order of the things remembered. I remember, for example, the deafening roar that went up when the Royal Family appeared on the balcony of the palace and the even greater roar when Churchill joined them there. Some time later, I remember the lights going on in their thousands, illuminating the public buildings and monuments of London. Nelson's Column, Admiralty Arch, the National Gallery, and the palace itself glowed rose red in the new found light: they can never have looked more beautiful. There were fireworks galore and to the north, in the direction of Hampstead, the night sky was alight with flickering bonfires. Searchlights swept overhead at random and then, miraculously, came together in a giant cone. Torches flared in the sconces outside the clubs of St James's and Pall Mall. London, after six years of stygian darkness, was luxuriating in an orgy of light.

How, or even if, I got home that night is uncertain. My flatmate, from whom I became separated in the mêlée, is equally uncertain about his movements and for the same reasons. What I do know is that in the course of whatever went on, and wherever it happened, I lost my forage cap, which in cruder parlance enjoys a cruder name. Be this as it may, the events of that incredible day are recorded, albeit negatively, by virtue of the absence of the aforementioned cap from my uniform, which our local clothes museum seemed delighted to have when, a few years ago, I had a clear out of inessential jumble.

Incidentally, should anyone, by some remote chance, have retained my cap as a memento, would they kindly return it. It is clearly marked,

100483 H R ROLLIN W/Cdr.

Famine

HUGH SINCLAIR

The famine in the western Netherlands was unique. It started abruptly on 17 September 1944 when Professor Gerbrandy, Prime Minister of the Netherlands government exiled in London, authorised a broadcast by the BBC to the Dutch people almost all of whom had in their homes illicit wireless receivers; they were asked immediately to paralyse all transport by a general railway strike. This the Dutch did with their customary efficiency. The unexpressed purpose was to hamper the movements of Nazi troops when, on that day, the airborne attack on Arnhem was launched. After that heroic failure through some extraordinary oversight the Dutch were not told to stop the paralysis of transport. The western Netherlands is mainly towns, water, and bulbs; and the Reich's kommissar, Seyss-Inquart, informed the Dutch authorities that a serious famine would result unless the railways operated again. The Dutch held their ground and an embargo on food from the northern and eastern occupied areas resulted. Quickly the per caput ration fell to 400 calories a day; mortality rose dramatically.

Early in 1945 steps were taken in London to deal as soon as practical with this serious situation. A major part was played by Sir Jack Drummond of the Ministry of Food; Professor H P (later Sir Harold) Himsworth of the Medical Research Council; Dr Virgil Sydenstricker (who had come from being professor of medicine in Augusta, Georgia, in 1942 to help the war effort and spent much time with my group centred in Oxford); and Dr Charles Leach of the Rockefeller Foundation (who had had personal experience of starvation). In order rapidly to assess the nutritional situation upon liberation and advise on relief, three nutrition survey teams were formed: one under Wing Commander Jack McCreary of the RCAF, one under Dr Fredrick Stare of Harvard, and a third from my group – the Oxford Nutrition Survey – which had been working for Sir Wilson Jameson of the Ministry of Health since early in the war.

Gas, electricity, and chemicals were mainly unavailable in occupied Holland, and therefore we decided to build and equip two mobile laboratories. Though Himsworth telephoned me on 26 March 1945 to say we would not be able to take transport to Holland, I had already contacted Lord Nuffield, who gave all assistance at Morris Motors. We received a Ford van on 9 April and a Dennis van the following day; on this day Drummond informed me that we could take two vans. Three days later Baird & Tatlock Ltd offered immediate help with equipment. The Dennis was completely converted and equipped (generator with voltage stabiliser, x ray machine, calor gas, laboratory benches) by 24 April (14 days after delivery) and the Ford the following day (16 days). I had flown to Holland with Drummond a little earlier (18 April), spending three days making arrangements for the Oxford Nutrition Survey team: Brian Lloyd as biochemist, Charlotte Wood as dietitian who also did venepunctures and measurements of dark adaptation, Vincent Quinn for haematology and various other jobs, and Keith Taylor for biochemical estimations. The vans left for Holland with my team on 3 May and I flew there the following day. We had an arrangement with the Nazi high command through the International Red Cross to get in before liberation, but in fact news of this arrived on the evening of 4 May.

We had already had experience of nutritional problems in Holland since, as the Allies advanced and liberated areas, Dutch paediatricians selected the worst nourished children who were flown to camps in this country and immediately examined by the Oxford Nutrition Survey staff. There were 485 children from Maastricht at a camp at Coventry in February 1945, 497 from 9 towns at Hull in March, and 267 from camps subsequently. The examination in general included clinical evaluation (with slit lamp examination of the eye), measurement of dark adaptation, and a variety of estimations on a sample of blood. The clinical examination, together with measurements of weight, height, and thickness of subcutaneous tissue revealed – as expected from the method of selection in Holland – that undernutrition was a serious problem especially in the 8–12 year age group.

It would probably have been easier in wartime to transport two Churchill tanks from Oxford to Holland than two mobile laboratories with civilians, since they did not fit military regulations in Supreme Headquarters Allied Expeditionary Force (SHAEF). But the Department of Social Affairs of the Netherlands government in London and Lady Falmouth of the British Red Cross could not have been more helpful over all the problems: movement orders, petrol, vaccinations, all documents (including laboratory instructions) to pass the censor, battledress, toilet paper, and derestriction of curfew. Most documents were required in quintuplicate but there had to be seven copies of all reports. Once the vans had arrived they got lost and while they were being traced I had the opportunity, with Virgil Sydenstricker, to make a rapid assessment of the situation. Of course in towns we first called on the mayor and the senior public health official. But this was on and a few days after liberation, when many officials were rapidly removed because they had collaborated with the Nazis.

On Saturday 5 May and Monday 7 May Sydenstricker and I motored to various towns and made contact with the Netherlands Military Administration (NMA) the head of which was Major General Kruls. The Sunday was spent in Belsen with Colonel Johnson who was in charge of medical arrangements. Here, as elsewhere, protein hydrolysates were being used. Drummond in particular had been impressed by allegations that in the Bengal famine starving persons could not digest protein. Therefore, at enormous cost, protein hydrolysates (by acid or enzymatic) were produced from casein (except in the case of one firm from meat). They were repulsive to drink and caused thrombosis if given intravenously. Starving persons want the food to which they are accustomed and in general have no difficulty in digesting large amounts. The exception was a mental hospital in Arnhem where, by some miracle of devotion, the nuns had kept the incontinent patients spotlessly clean despite no soap or hot water; here the ravenous inmates drank litres of the nauseous stuff.

Angry exchanges

Tuesday 8 May was VE Day, though we hardly noticed this, and Sydenstricker and I had to visit NMA and then go to Leiden where I had decided to set up my headquarters. We were in a hurry and our Dutch driver knew a short cut across country. At the end of a large field we met an irate British regular army colonel suitably reinforced with miscellaneous personnel. He stopped us, swore at us, and informed us we had been motoring through a heavily mined area. Sydenstricker, a typically courteous soft spoken Georgian gentleman, and I both had acquired rank of full colonel, I just turned 35 years old and he nearly twice my age, so our mean age nearly matched our adversary and we were two colonels against one. In retrospect I have wondered how that paragon of military etiquette, Elston Grey-Turner, would have handled the situation; he was a born leader of men, inevitably the senior prefect at Winchester and then president of the Cambridge University Medical Society and of the Abernethian Society at Barts; and sitting opposite him for years on the Court of the Apothecaries, I never so far as I recall voted differently from his lead. As I had been brought up with a regular army father and elder brother, I did not have the same respect for military etiquette. My polite suggestion that we must have overlooked some notice stating "Beware of mines" did not appeal to the colonel, nor did my observation that we had survived, which was a matter for rejoicing rather than abuse. Anyhow, we were in a hurry, had valid movement orders, and intended to proceed. Sydenstricker said nothing, but as soon as we had disentangled ourselves from the army he amazed me by cursing the innocent driver; we had worked together in various difficult circumstances, I had always admired his courtesy towards everyone, and I had never before seen him unjustifiably angry.

A few days later, however, both he and I could hardly control our righteous rage. Major General Warren Draper, who had been US deputy surgeon general and was in charge of the public health branch of SHAEF, had on occasion visited me in Oxford during the war; now he motored through liberated Holland and made a press release which *The Times* published on 23 May: "We expected to find the most terrible conditions there, but we did not need the special teams which stood by ready for action. There were some cases of advanced malnutrition, but no cases of actual starvation." Starving persons dying in their beds do not go out in the streets to wave flags at a scurrying major general, and Sydenstricker and I sent a furious letter to *The Times* to say so, but it was politely declined to preserve Allied accord.

In fact, some 10 000 persons are estimated to have died from actual starvation in the acute famine in the Netherlands. Our team, unwanted by Draper but not by the Dutch, operated mainly by examining some 3500 persons in Leiden and The Hague where we were given streets in different social areas by the public health authorities and selected every tenth house. The occupants were requested all to visit our clinic, where they were thoroughly investigated; but a social worker visited each house so that we could go to examine those too ill to visit us. Our team was joined by a great many liberated Dutch scientists, including the sons of Professor B C P Jansen of Amsterdam and Professor Kuenen of Leiden, and the staff of Dr van Eekelen (who himself had lost 50lb) the director of the Central Institute for Food Research in Utrecht; the professor of biochemistry, Bungeburg de Jong, himself suffering from starvation, put his department in Leiden at our disposal, and help was provided by Dr Dekker, conservator of Medische Chemie. We did some 25 000 biochemical estimations in a few weeks. One problem was the cause of the prevalent famine oedema. We estimated protein in plasma by five methods: gravimetric, biuret, micro-Kjeldahl, densitometric (Linderstrøm-Lang) and copper sulphate (Van Slyke); we also estimated it in oedema fluid. The oedema was not caused by low colloid osmotic pressure of plasma as Starling had proposed. Since nutrition was rapidly improving as foods were flown in, we thought we would collect a small sample of hair from the head and estimate amino acids along it. During the first day our workers obtained no hair: collaborators with the Nazis had their hair shaved (and some were made to clean pavements with toothbrushes), so the request for a small sample of hair was misinterpreted until we realised the problem and carefully explained the reason.

Magnificent race

The Ministry of Health in London was delighted at the success of the test it had introduced for assessing the nutritional state of children. A broom handle of specified diameter was placed across a door and corner of a room, and the time measured for which a child could hang by the arms. We found, amazingly, that two children hanging together were much better nourished than either alone, and the Dutch children severely undernourished: the bar test came at the end of a long examination including venepucture, and they knew that when they dropped off they would receive the award of chocolate, something of which they had heard but had not tasted. They did not hang for long.

Whenever I visited a leading clinician or public health official I was never asked for food or cigarettes; the former had been in very short supply and was supplemented with tulip bulbs (daffodil bulbs were toxic), and cigarettes were unobtainable – but I always took a packet of 20 and carelessly left it behind. Even the magnificent medical scholar Professor Groen, when he came into my clinic in Leiden, said he had come from Amsterdam hearing allied doctors had arrived and asked if he could watch our work, but did not mention that he had been hiding in a cellar for 14 days without food. The treatment by the Dutch of the former occupying force was immaculate: they disarmed the Nazis, pointed the way to Germany, and completely ignored them as privates and generals alike walked dejectedly home. The Dutch are a magnificent race.

Change in the air

DEREK STEVENSON

London, where I had spent the last three years of the war, was in 1945 a very different city from the one we know today. The onslaught of the blitz in 1941 and 1942, and later the violent impact of Hitler's secret weapons, the V1 and the V2, had indiscriminately destroyed so many of the buildings and familiar landmarks that even a Londoner could be excused for losing himself in the changed surroundings. Instead of today's tourists, Americans, Germans, and Japanese – all seemingly young, dressed alike in denim, and carrying cameras – the city, though just as crowded, was then totally peopled by men and women in uniform, the ubiquitous gas mask replacing the camera.

It seemed as if all those nations which had responded to the call for freedom were represented on the streets of the city. Czechs, Poles, Free French, Dutch, Americans, and Belgians, all in their distinctive uniforms, all making their way to Whitehall where the cheering crowds lined the streets to applaud the chief architect of victory, Winston Churchill, who, standing on the balcony of the old Ministry of Health building, delighted all by his beaming smile and his victory sign.

An end to all things military

Although the day had been declared a public holiday it was business as usual at the War Office, where I was then working as a staff officer to the director general in the army medical directorate. Indeed, only the day before I had received a terse message from the Secretary of State for War indicating that the Prime Minister himself had "prayed" that at least 2000 doctors be released from the army and returned to civilian life within the next four weeks.

151

Somewhat bemused by this, I hastily sought out my chief and inquired whether he thought that the message should be taken seriously. After all, our medical officers were scattered over the four corners of the earth, communications and transportation were difficult, and the war against Japan had yet to be won. Moreover, I detected the subtle hand of Lord Moran, personal physician to Mr Churchill, with whom he had not a little influence on medical matters.

How naive can you be at the age of 32?

I was quickly and firmly told that it was not for me to question the workings of higher authority, but, to use current vernacular, to "get on my bike" and ensure that the instructions were promptly put in hand. That immediate effect was given to the Prime Minister's "prayer" was a tribute not to any excessive zeal or expertise on my part but to the combined determination of service men and women, and their dependents at home, to put an end to all things military and ensure an early return to civilian life after five long years of separation. Indeed the Prime Minister's intervention illustrated vividly the constant struggle that had gone on from the outset of war between those who supported the insatiable demand of the armed forces for more and more doctors, and those who believed that the civilian medical services were already cut to the bone, and that air raid casualties in the United Kingdom were equally deserving of prompt medical attention.

During the phoney war of 1939–40, and later on when our forces were being reassembled for the invasion of Europe, this conflict of views assumed emotive proportions, and it was frequently claimed that doctors in uniform were having an easy privileged time, whereas their counterparts in civilian life, without the glamour of uniform, were carrying what was fast becoming an unacceptable burden. But all this was quickly forgotten on VE Day when the whole nation paused in its united endeavour, to celebrate not only a great victory against great odds, but a task which could only have been achieved by a wholly united people.

Behind the rejoicing

Already, however, it was possible to detect a change in the political thinking of those very people who were totally behind their leaders and in particular the Prime Minister himself. With the end of the war in Europe in sight, tempers in parliament were on a knife edge, and it was becoming increasingly clear that the national government had finally served its useful purpose. Already the bitterness of party politics had begun to assert itself, and the clamour for a speedy general election grew in intensity. Behind the natural rejoicing on VE Day, and in the months to follow, it was possible to detect that a dramatic change in the lifestyle of the country was approaching. A number of factors were to play their part: the publication of the Beveridge Report with its plan for a welfare state to cater for all from the cradle to the grave, and its clear indication that the lynchpin of this welfare state would need to be a comprehensive national health service; the strongly held views of returning service men and women that after six years of war the old order of class and privilege was no longer acceptable, and that this time the unemployment and discontent which followed in the wake of World War I would not be tolerated.

Perhaps it was necessary to be at the heart of events to appreciate the subtle way in which the need for change was brought to the notice of service men and women. Certainly every opportunity was taken in the steady stream of educative booklets issued to the troops by the army bureau of current affairs. Be that as it may, on VE Day change was in the air. A discerning observer might sense that the vast crowds of people were determined that this time the sacrifices made would be vindicated by a new and better world to which their relatives and friends would shortly be returning.

But what of the spirit of the nation in 1945? No one who lived through those wartime years could have failed to be heartened by the strength of common purpose, the loyalty to a common cause – the defeat of Hitler and all he stood for – and the universal sense of humour, and all this despite rigorous food rationing and total blackout. It would have been rash for anyone to bet on that day that Mr Churchill was shortly to suffer overwhelming defeat at the polls. His standing in the country was demonstrated on VE Day by almost mass hysteria, and few could have predicted the landslide defeat which was to happen in so short a time. That happening, it could be argued, proved beyond all doubt that when change is sought people will always vote for policies and not personalities.

History will probably record VE Day as a watershed in the affairs of Great Britain. Within a few years, the British Empire, whose representatives could be seen everywhere on the streets of the capital city, would disappear and be replaced by a loose Commonwealth of Nations. The era of atomic fission was about to break with all its fearsome consequences for the future. Five years of socialist administration were to change the face of Great Britain, and our wartime ally, Russia, was to expand its territory in eastern Europe and menace the free world.

Tomorrow, just you wait and see

It is doubtful if much of this was uppermost in the minds of those attending the victory celebrations throughout the country. The sense of relief at the cessation of hostilities in Europe was too great. In 1945 London was the free capital city of the free world. Londoners walked tall. National pride overshadowed party politics. Church bells, silenced for so long, pealed out their message of hope for all, and on the night of VE Day the lights, switched on all over the city, somehow symbolised the heart of the people.

It was a day, and night, I can never forget.

Where next?

T D V SWINSCOW

Cries of joy and triumph and laughter swelled from the town square of Newark-on-Trent (where we were stationed) as I walked towards it on the evening of 8 May 1945. For them it was really over at last, the European and most immediately threatening part of the war, and they were celebrating the lifting of a frightful burden. But reminded by the distant laughter through the dusk of friends who had been killed I turned back before ever reaching the crowds and went over to the officers' mess, the only home I had known, in various places and units, for the past four years. Several of the officers were there, and we continued discussing a topic that had already displaced the impulse to enjoy a carefree celebration – where next?

We knew that VE Day had not brought the end of the war for us in the 1st Airborne Reconnaissance Squadron. It could only be a pause before the next operation, perhaps in Europe, perhaps in Japan. Rumour had it that despite the armistice on Lüneburg Heath the Germans would try to continue the war in the mountains of Scandinavia and Austria. Having already taken part in two invasions – by sea at Algiers in 1942 and by parachute at Arnhem in 1944 – I felt a degree of professional curiosity as we discussed the possibilities. All of us were in our twenties, and warfare was the only occupation most of us had known in adult life, except for my six months as a house surgeon after qualifying. The war had become our life. It had brought us adventure, boredom, excitement, grief, and, especially in the 1st Airborne Division, an unforgettable sense of trust and comradeship – something that Elston Grey-Turner would have especially appreciated. In the continuity of this experience VE Day was but a ripple.

Intense relief

As a medical man I fell to reflecting on some of the experiences I had had. Two in particular came into my mind, probably because they made my role seem strikingly, reassuringly worthwhile in a world of horror and pain. Early in 1943 in Tunisia I was on a hot, hard, dusty hillside as medical officer to a group of advanced army headquarters intelligence units intercepting and decoding the enemy's radio messages. A few German planes suddenly appeared on a bombing raid. One of the casualties of the raid was a soldier brought to my aid post in terrible agony from burns of his body, his face blackened, hair charred, and uniform in tatters. Here I remembered advice given to me when I was a student: in emergency don't hesitate to give morphine intravenously. The soldier was a tall man of powerful physique, so I decided on the large dose of $\frac{1}{2}$ grain (32 mg) and injected it very slowly into an arm vein. The effect was instantaneous and wonderful, and to this day I can see the expression of pure bliss into which his features relaxed as the opiate flowed into him. He made a good recovery.

Every doctor must at some time have felt the satisfaction of giving his patient such intense relief, and during the battle at Arnhem I had another experience of a similar kind. I was running to a house where I had set up an aid post, when I met a glider pilot wandering in the woods with a severe wound of his face. Most of his lower jaw had been shot away, and he soon made plain to me in sign language that he was parched with thirst, for the wound had left him unable to drink, and wounded men generally suffer from thirst anyway. So I went to a nearby house and borrowed a teapot, filled it with water, and with some help from the wounded man himself managed to quench his thirst by slowly pouring the water from the spout into his gullet. Again, I can never forget the expression of blissful gratitude with which he thanked me for this small service. It haunts me to this day.

Narrow escapes

War's ugly face had also glared at me quite closely on several occasions. On one of them there was a little hillside outside Arnhem going down to a stream and then a slope up the other side to a wood. One of our men had been shot and had fallen on the hillside, so I ran out to attend to him, as the stretcher bearers were at that moment engaged elsewhere. But finding myself under fire from a machine gunner I threw myself down in the heather. Then a man with a mortar in the wood opposite saw his chance and put a mortar bomb six feet in front of me. No sooner had it exploded than I heard the plop of another bomb leaving the barrel, and it exploded six feet behind me. Then came another to one side at the same distance, and the thought occurred to me (probably as a defensive mechanism): could I see these bombs in flight, as I had heard was possible? Hearing another plop from the mortar barrel I looked up straining to see the bomb, but there was only empty sky, and that bomb then exploded on the other side of me. An inevitable speculation now entered my mind: would he hit the central point at which I lay? A fifth bomb joined the little circle, and then a sixth completed the clock face. Suddenly I realised no more were coming. I had been deliberately shot at six times – and missed. (A visitor to that spot in recent years has told me the bomb craters are still just visible in the heathland.) Now a stretcher bearer joined me from another direction, we reached our man, and picked him up. But the machine gunner sprayed us again, and one of the bullets broke up on the aluminium stretcher, giving another serious wound to the casualty and driving two splinters into my back on either side of the spinal cord, just missing it by a few millimetres. Fate had been kind to me. And so it was again two nights later, when I woke at dawn after sleeping crouched in a slit trench to find, actually lying across its edge within a few inches of my head, a German 105 mm shell that had failed to explode – or even to wake me when it landed.

Strange incident

Ours was an odd existence, I reflected, as we discussed "Where next?" – a life composed of order and anarchy, with its expectation of the unexpected, its realisation of the unimaginable. If a town stood in our way, bomb it; if a building, blow it up; if a man, kill him; if women and children . . . but there was still a point at which our hearts were touched. And the next day we had the answer to our question of where next: Norway! So we "stood to" and then we were off – for me the third time I was to land at war among strangers.

After an alarming flight through low cloud over the North Sea we landed at Stavanger. One plane crashed in the mountains on that flight (like surgical operations, military operations have a death rate). The Germans had about 200 000 troops in Norway, mostly of poor quality. We were outnumbered more than 100 to one, but in these circumstances numbers counted for much less than the confidence that animated us and the dejection that weighed in the enemy's heart. The show of strength was enough, and the German command there fell into line with the armistice agreement. Our task evolved into hunting down Gestapo agents and SS troops.

Now I had another odd experience, for this proved to be the only time in the war when I was taken prisoner by the Germans – if briefly. We had landed at an airfield some miles south of Stavanger, and I wanted to get into the town to discover what medical facilities it had. To my surprise I saw a German staff car driving towards the town, so I stepped out and halted it. An officer and driver were inside. Accompanied by one of our unit's officers armed with an automatic pistol I ordered the Germans to take us into Stavanger. They appeared to agree, but in fact drove us off into a nearby fairy tale castle (it had been built originally for a film) complete with drawbridge, portcullis, and castellated walls. Arrived in the castle's courtyard, and surrounded by German soldiers with (it seemed odd to me at the time) fixed bayonets, I could do little but get out and demand to see the commanding officer. He proved to be a pleasant and genial man with a sense of humour, so I explained to him that I wished to be driven into Stavanger on medical business. He said, "You have no right to stop my vehicles," to which I replied, "You have lost the war." This went on for some time, but he was reasonable in defeat and I was probably unreasonable in victory. He let me and my fellow officer go in his staff car to Stavanger.

Signatures to history

Apart from this little exchange the operation in Norway amounted to the joyful liberation of an oppressed and brave nation. But, as on VE Day, I did later have the impression again that the war was not really over and in a sense never would be. During an August afternoon I was sitting alone in a forest hut by Lake Mjøsa north of Oslo listening to the BBC news on a German radio set. As I tuned in the announcer startled me by describing the dropping of an atomic bomb on Hiroshima. This must be the end of warfare as I have known it, was my first thought – too sanguine as events have shown. And then I felt only a sense of relief that my warfaring days were nearing the end. So, when it came, VJ Day meant no more to me than VE Day: neither brought anything more than signatures to a history that had been made. For a time I sat in the silent wood in the filtered light of the spruce trees, feeling the presence of my friends who had been killed in the war – most of the friends of my youth – just as the memory of them had troubled my mind when I turned away from the crowds on VE Day. Life had to be lived, and I have put the shadows away from me, but I felt then, and still feel, an immeasurable debt.

> Friends of my youth, a last adieu!
>   haply some day we meet again;
> Yet ne'er the self-same men shall meet;
>   the years shall make us other men.
> The light of morn has grown to noon,
>   has paled to eve, and now farewell!
> Go, vanish from my life as dies
>   the tinkling of the camel's bell.
>   – *Sir Richard Burton.*

Passage to India

SELWYN TAYLOR

To recall VE Day at all I have to think furiously, where was I? what was I doing? But an invitation to do honour to Elston Grey-Turner is a pleasant task and I immediately conjure up a picture of him in his master's robes welcoming his guests at the top of the staircase at the Society of Apothecaries. I owe a double debt to his family because I was asked by his father to send for his old patients for follow up at Hammersmith – and on these occasions he really did put his bowler hat over the teapot to keep it warm in sister's office, as Sister Tawse's eyes twinkled appreciatively. He was very wise and particularly helpful to me.

I was stationed in Mombasa on VE Day, and since it was declared a holiday we had a very good lunch. I also recall shooting at a vulture with my old 16 bore in the afternoon – the bird left in disgust and unharmed. On such an auspicious day my social conscience constrained me to invite Matron to the wardroom for dinner. In those days we changed every evening and in short white dress jacket with stripes on shoulder, black tie, cummerbund, and black trousers it was indeed rather a smart turnout. A tropical evening, an excellent meal, and because I had travelled out via South Africa (where I had done a course in tropical medicine with the high and low Gears in Johannesburg) we imbibed that delicious digestif half Van Der Hum/half brandy with our coffee. The weekly film show followed and was the usual American musical, I quite forget which; we held hands in that velvety warm darkness which you only find in the tropics. When I awoke, everyone had left. Yes, I was desperately embarrassed, but youth is made of resilient stuff and I didn't actually have to meet Matron next day.

Decision in Tavistock Square

I always associate Elston with BMA House and it was indeed in that very building that my future career was inadvertently shaped. I had qualified in June 1939, but when war broke out our senior staff at King's moved into the residents' quarters and the house job I was about to take up no longer existed. I'd always promised myself I would make no further financial demands on my parents as soon as I was qualified; indeed I hoped to repay something, as the thirties had been a time of great financial depression and a country schoolmaster is not an affluent member of society. Needing a job I went back to Oxford, thinking I might be a demonstrator of anatomy for I needed more experience in that field to sit for my primary, and my old moral tutor had now retired to Bradmore Road with his sister and would certainly give me a bed. Walking down the Cornmarket I met the professor – Le Gros Clark – and asked him what chance there was, as term started later that week. He could not have been more friendly (I had previously worked under him as a junior), but unfortunately all the paid posts were now filled; he thought, however, that I might be gainfully employed if I appeared on the first day of term. This I did, and all the pupils needing tutorials who could not be taken by Alice Carleton or the other staff were passed on to me. I was suddenly so rich that the following week I proposed marriage and in October took the most intelligent step of my life. We found a minute flat in Norham Gardens and soon after, when term ended, were both summoned to work in the newly set up Emergency Medical Service.

Down at Horton Hospital near Epsom, previously a vast semi-circular mental establishment, working day and night on the casualties from Europe – especially after Dunkirk – I realised that if I stayed on I should one day be conscripted into the RAMC, and as I had a consuming passion for the sea I wanted to serve in the navy. I therefore made an appointment at BMA House to interview the secretary, a predecessor of Elston, who proved to be Charles Hill, his voice familiar as the "Radio Doctor". I explained that I now had the primary, was working for the final FRCS in the EMS, but wished to join the navy. In avuncular manner he told me that I would be of much more use in the war effort as a well trained surgeon, that I should stay where I was, obtain the FRCS and, yes, I would almost inevitably be recruited into the army. I thanked him, walked down the corridor and forthwith signed on for the navy.

It was, for me, the right choice and indeed the shortage of ships meant that I was not sent for until October 1940, on the very anniversary of our wedding, to go to Portsmouth. In due course, with two wavy stripes, I reported and also told the PMO that I had applied to take the final FRCS in two weeks' time. He was most helpful and said that I could certainly have leave to sit for it.

Friendly advice

When my examination card arrived the venue had been changed from Queen Square, London, to the Queen Elizabeth Hospital, Birmingham, because of the air raids on London; the college in Lincoln's Inn Fields was not hit until May, 1941. I stayed with Quaker in-laws at Bournville, there was bible reading at breakfast, and it was a delightful oasis in those anxious times. The papers were to my liking and we were told that candidates in uniform would be given their vivas first thing next morning so that they could return to their units, but when I reached Bournville in the evening a telegram awaited me: "Report forthwith to Liverpool to await posting". My adoptive uncle was a splendid character; seeing how crestfallen I was, he slid the telegram under the blotting pad on the hall table and said, "Now if it had fallen there you would have missed seeing it. I suggest you finish the examination tomorrow morning and then go to Liverpool." Of course that is just what I did, but had to leave before the results were announced and security forbade my saying what my address would be.

I stayed at the Adelphi Hotel and days later I headed out in a small boat into the November murk beyond the Royal Liver building to a bedraggled V & W destroyer of World War 1 vintage just back from two weeks' convoy duties in the north Atlantic. As I climbed aboard, saluting the quarterdeck, the captain came aft and called out, "Welcome aboard, doc. I understand that I have to congratulate you on becoming a fellow of the Royal College of Surgeons." So that was why I was serving as a surgical specialist in Mombasa on VE Day.

What was I doing? Well, there was a modest flow of surgical problems to deal with and very congenial colleagues to help solve them. I remember being very excited when I diagnosed and drained a perinephric abscess in a sailor brought in from the

162

Seychelles with pyrexia of unknown origin. I also recall the sadness when, after flying to Zanzibar – in those days it was like a page straight out of the Arabian Nights – I failed to save a patient with a massive amoebic liver abscess. The African continent is a most beguiling mistress and I still feel the tug to return even after 40 years. Leave up country in Kenya was glorious and the plants, the trees, and the game entrancing. In Mombasa we had to pursue our own intellectual refreshment; the American consul was particularly kind after I operated on his volatile French wife and he used to pass on to me their medical information sheets. Thus it was I first read about the Blalock–Taussig operation and almost doubted its feasibility. We started a little literary society: I remember Edward Lowbury the poet was pathologist at the nearby army hospital, there was a judge whom we made chairman, and an East African Railways official who contributed much. The rule was that we each gave a paper; mine was entitled "Rhyme without reason" and my tastes do not appear to have changed significantly 40 years on.

Within weeks we had packed up hospital and headed east to Bombay in a British India Steam Navigation ship to regroup for operation "Zipper" and the landings in Malaya.

Before and after

STEPHEN TAYLOR

The second world war crept up on us gradually, with none of the hysterical excitement which marked the commencement of the 1914–18 war. This unimpressive beginning in 1939 was followed by months of suspended animation, the so called "phoney war", before things really started to move. A similar contrast was exhibited by their two endings. November 11, 1918, the eleventh hour of the eleventh day of the eleventh month, was a moment of intense drama. The senseless slaughter was ended at last and everyone, or almost everyone, burst into spontaneous rejoicing. VE Day, on the other hand, was not a climax. We knew it was all over bar the shouting long before the final shot was fired.

I had spent most of the war as director of home intelligence at the Ministry of Information. It was my job to record as accurately as possible for the government the state of civilian morale and public opinion. By 1941 we had learnt our job and become reasonably efficient. Each Thursday morning our weekly report was circulated to the Cabinet and about 200 other top officials telling them what the British public was thinking and feeling during the week ending the previous Monday. These reports are now in the public domain and are available to all at the new Public Record Office at Kew. The Germans also had a home intelligence department, but when its reports became increasingly gloomy it was suppressed and its director dismissed.

In a way, we suffered a similar fate, but for a more honourable reason. In December 1944 the powers that be (in fact the late Sir Cyril Radcliffe) decided that the home intelligence weekly reports should cease, as the war was virtually over, and public opinion could express itself well enough through the normal channels. In one sense this was a wrong decision, since we had repeatedly shown that parliament and the press were very inaccurate reflectors of public opinion. By and large, public opinion was far more down to earth and unexcitable than either of these two indicators. But both were jealous of their functions and could be expected to attack the Ministry of Information increasingly for intrusion into their spheres. Moreover, some intelligence work was already showing an increasingly anti–Conservative swing in opinion, and we might have found ourselves in the centre of a political row. So perhaps Sir Cyril was, on balance, right after all. None of us in the department minded, as we all had other fish to fry.

Marker on the road to peace

I can best show how VE Day was for the general public at home only a marker on the road to peace by a brief chronology. With the fighting forces it may well have been different.

6 June 1944. D Day. Allied invasion of Normandy.

13 June 1944. First flying bombs (V1s) fell on Britain. As "morale busters" these were never a serious threat.

25 August 1944. Paris liberated.

3 September 1944. Brussels liberated.

8 September 1944. First rocket bombs (V2s) fell on Britain, with even less effect than the V1s.

17 September 1944. Blackout ended. Part time civil defence workers released. Home Guard call up ended and compulsory drills stopped.

28 April 1945. Link up of the American and Russian troops on the River Elbe.

2 May 1945. Suicide of Hitler announced. Whitehall issued *Guide to Celebrations at the End of the War with Germany*.

4 May 1945. At 6.21 pm all the German armies in north west Germany, Denmark, and Holland surrendered unconditionally to Field Marshal Montgomery's Twenty first Army Group, the surrender to be effective at 8 am on 5 May.

8 May 1945. We celebrated VE Day.

The Germans had been trying desperately to surrender *all* their forces to the Western Allies rather than to the Russians, but we would have none of it. On 9 May, they surrendered formally and unconditionally to all the Allies in Berlin.

There was some public rejoicing, some street parties, and flags left over from the last war were produced, but it was a very restrained affair. The end of the war in Europe did not mean the end of clothes rationing or food rationing or furniture rationing, or the housing shortage. Rather did it mean that we faced the biggest uphill struggle in our history, which to some extent is still going on.

On 23 May 1945, the wartime coalition government came to an end, and Mr Churchill formed a caretaker Conservative government to carry on until a general election could be held. He wanted to keep the coalition in operation until the end of the war with Japan, but the Labour party would not hear of it. They were proved right, for policy differences about postwar reconstruction were so deep that a new start was essential. So on 5 July a general election was held, the first for 10 years, and the first in which many millions of new voters took part.

Turning point

On 27 April it was announced that Dr Stephen Taylor had been selected as prospective parliamentary candidate by the local Labour party for the constituency of Barnet. I knew very little of the machinery of practical politics. I did not know, for example, that Barnet was regarded as one of the safest Conservative seats in the country, and I had never a moment's doubt that I would win. I was already slightly in the public eye, for in December 1944 Mr Herbert Morrison had spoken at a public luncheon to launch a book I had written called *Battle for Health*. It was the first of a series called *The New Democracy*, and in a few weeks it had sold its full print of 15 000 copies.

Herbert Morrison was Home Secretary at the time, and had announced his decision that there should be a woman to govern Holloway Prison. The post was publicly advertised, and my wife, Dr Charity Taylor, who was at that time junior medical officer at the prison, decided to apply. She was, I believe, the youngest applicant, among a distinguished collection of her seniors.

Things dragged on, and once I became a Labour candidate at the election it was important, to avoid any charges of favouritism and a bad start to her term of office if she got the job, that she should if possible be appointed by a Conservative Home Secretary. This meant that the decision and the announcement had to be made between 23 May, when the Conservative caretaker government took over, and 26 July, when the election results were announced. She just made it: her appointment as the first woman governor of Holloway Prison was made by the Conservative Home Secretary, Sir Donald Sommervell, on 18 July 1945. If the count for the general election had not been delayed for 13 days, to allow all the services votes to come in, things might have turned out differently. I got in by a 682 vote majority over my opponent, Sir Andrew Clark KC, who had been widely tipped as the next Attorney General. As the policeman said at the polling station, "If Barnet's gone red, Britain's gone red".

The end of the war and the July 1945 election marked a turning point in the lives of all of us. Things would never be the same again. For the great majority of us, and on balance, it was a turning point for the better. It is good to have seen real poverty abolished, good health care for all established, an end to the housing shortage, and food and clothes and consumer goods in plenty for all. But there is still much to be done. We do not yet know how to deal with the hysterical psychopaths in positions of power. We do not know how to cure what Professor John Ryle called "the great pandemic of our time – fear". But we did much better in 1945 than in 1918, and that fact alone ought to give us a glimmer of hope for the future.

Some reflections on the class of '45

JOHN WALTON

What on earth *did* I do on VE Day? Some memories, but regrettably few, are crystal clear; others are swathed in mist so obscure that concentration achieves no clarity; and yet others are so vague and imprecise that it would be injudicious to commit them to paper for fear of contradiction. I do know that I was a final year medical student, hopefully about to qualify, working in dear Elston's beloved native city where his distinguished father had adorned the department of surgery before his translation to Hammersmith. So perhaps it would be appropriate in 1984, when the alumni of the Newcastle Medical School celebrate the 150th anniversary of its foundation as a constituent part of the University of Durham, if my hazy recollections included not only something about the day itself but also about that school and the university which conferred upon Elston an honorary doctorate of medicine during the BMA Annual Representative Meeting of 1980.

Learning quickly

On VE Day itself I was completing my midwifery clerking at the Princess Mary Maternity Hospital, where some eight of us lived in a decaying hut with thin plasterboard partitions. There were several holes in the wall of the solitary bathroom so that the female houseman who shared it was compelled to drape articles of clothing over these apertures in order to achieve privacy. After three or four weeks at the PMMH we had all overcome our initial shock and apprehension on learning (when qualified resident staff were very few) that all anaesthetics for deliveries were to be given by us students. We worked by rota, often around the clock, and inevitably learned quickly.

When a call came to go out on "the district", two students went by taxi to collect the obstetric bag at Jubilee Road and then carried on, either by taxi or by bicycle, to the patient's home. Usually a midwife was available, but not always, and sometimes one of a frightened pair of students in Byker would retire to the lavatory with a copy of "Eden and Holland" before emerging to offer whispered instructions to his partner. We were instructed to telephone the RSO if something exceptional turned up, but occasionally he could not be contacted and I well remember the occasion when two of us, at first with mounting apprehension but subsequently with a sense of pride, managed a successful breech delivery. Even more alarming was the case of the patient with the brisk postpartum haemorrhage in the labour ward. After we had cross matched the blood and begun the transfusion, I, under the anxious gaze of a fellow student and a midwife, did a manual removal of placenta because the RSO was dealing with an emergency on the district and the one qualified houseman was doing a forceps delivery elsewhere.

Amidst all this intense activity, the tremendous sense of excitement and the pervasive sense of relief which so dominated our thoughts on VE Day were a little submerged by the pressing clinical responsibilities which came so early to us as final year students in time of war. But we did have an impromptu party in the hut, with some of the senior and established consultants, such as Stanley Way, flitting in and out and manufacturing potentially lethal beverages. Two enterprising students scoured Jesmond for sufficient wood to allow us the luxury of a bonfire, something denied to us throughout the long war years. Sadly, the fine rain of the afternoon and evening quelled the flames if not the enthusiasm. Some, not on duty, joined the capacity congregation at St Thomas's Church before going on to the splendid SRC dance in King's Hall. Some simply gazed in deep reflection upon the floodlighting of St Thomas's and Grey's monument and a city bedecked with flags awakening from its wartime drabness. But in the midst of all the rejoicing, the single most endearing memory is of the obvious relief, joy, and unadulterated happiness shown by the young Geordie mums and mothers to be in hospital as they recognised that at last their menfolk, many serving overseas or in the navy or merchant navy, were out of danger.

Quis custodiet?

Being a medical student in wartime brought many problems. Before and during the Battle of Britain many of us felt some guilt, as medical students, at being in a reserved occupation; some even failed examinations deliberately in order to join the forces. I well recall the wise counsel of the then dean, Professor R B Green, when he agreed at my entrance interview to release me after a year if I still persisted in my wish to join the RAF. He well recognised that once in the university one's interest in the work, in company with many others, made such conflicting loyalties in a country at war much easier to bear. Early in the war, in our first summer vacation, working as labourers on an airfield under construction in Norfolk helped a little. And of course we were all enrolled in the Senior Training Corps and paraded twice weekly in uniform on Wednesday afternoons and Saturday mornings.

Service in "the corps" brought many memorable experiences, not least that which occurred when Major General Philip Mitchener, DDMS Northern Command, came to inspect us. The inspection was followed by a marchpast along Queen Victoria Road. One of our officers, intending to lead his company to the rear of the medical school where they would enter to hear the general's lecture, suddenly found himself marching alone along the road because a student sergeant, with spirited independence, had given the "left wheel" from the rear of the squad and the troops had turned into the front entrance. And during one corps camp at Longhorsley the comments of our dean and CO, Lieutenant Colonel Green, were unrecordable when the CO of our host field ambulance called to pay his respects and elicited no reaction from the student on guard at the gate; as he subsequently argued cogently, the visiting dignitary did not look as if he wished to have the guard turned out.

One regular duty of the corps was to protect the medical school against air raids. Under an elaborate rota, every night 10 valiant students in the charge of a staff member were locked in the building with tin hats, stirrup pumps, sandbags, and other appropriate paraphernalia. The girls were not left out as some did rota duty on the telephone exchange in the main King's College building. Both groups soon discovered the system of underground heating tunnels which joined the basement of the medical school to King's, and access between the beleaguered centres was simple provided one knew the way. In the later years of the war when the blitz was a thing of the past, many squads developed a working arrangement whereby one or two people were left to hold the fort and others went to the cinema, with strict instructions to hurry back if the siren went. On one memorable occasion the organisation faltered and the entire squad arrived at the medical school after the show to find no student inside to open the door. Only the staff leader of the squad, Professor Dunlop, remained within in lonely splendour. Eventually he heard the clamour and opened up; being one of nature's gentlemen, he was most understanding.

Teachers and students

Professor Dunlop was also memorable for the mellifluous flow of English in which he delivered his lectures. Unfortunately their content was sometimes lost as the class waited breathlessly for the end of each sentence. But even in those wartime days, the quality of teaching was memorable. With nights on reception, assisting in the theatre, and ward rounds with dear Norman Hodgson, repeating again and again the cardinal signs of inflammation and the characteristics one must learn of every lump, knowledge slowly but surely grew. I remember especially the clear and logical ward teaching of Fred Nattrass, the virtuosity and brilliant inspiration of James Spence, and the dogmatism of Farquhar Murray in such striking contrast to the flamboyant but memorable obiter dicta of Harvey Evers. Harvey was most impressed when he came to lecture and found every male student in the class, like him, wearing his tie in a bow. And no one could possibly forget the sheer magnetism of Professor Arthur Frederick Bernard Shaw, autocrat of the department of pathology. When asked if he was any relation to *the* Bernard Shaw (his uncle) he said, "I *am the* Bernard Shaw". During our pathological clerking he closed the doors of the postmortem room at 9 am prompt and reopened them at 12.30 to release his captive student audience. About a dozen of us who worked at the central station as night porters for some two weeks or so over one Christmas vacation and then attended pathology clerking during the day were regularly shaken into reluctant wakefulness by the quality of his expositions and by the fearsome teaching of "Ginger" Thomson, then lecturer in pathology, subsequently professor in Cape Town.

Sadly, as we have learned when attending our five-yearly

171

reunions, 11 of our class of 80 who graduated in 1945 have died. Five hold, or have held, chairs, four in the USA and one in the UK; 15 are still practising in many specialties as consultants in the UK, and another six abroad; over 40 are in general practice, about two thirds of them in Northumberland, Durham, or North Yorkshire. Looking back, I doubt if we were very different from present day medical students; we were probably about as hard working (sporadically) and about as keen and conscientious as they are. Perhaps wartime and the clinical responsibility to which we were so quickly exposed as students helped us to mature a little earlier, but I doubt if the difference would stand statistical scrutiny. We could be rebellious against authority, vociferous in the defence of students' rights, and some were just as bawdy or boisterous or bibulous as are some students today. Frankly, the genus does not seem to have changed very much in the last 40 years, except that they now seem much younger; I wonder why?

Joy not unconfined

GORDON WOLSTENHOLME

One of my earliest memories is of Armistice Day 1918 when, perversely, I had a fight with a neighbouring boy over the size of our respective flags. Subsequently photographs and films of that day greatly intrigued me: what must it be like to celebrate with unconfined joy? Perhaps, when the second world war ended, I should find out.

But VE Day in Italy, when it came, found us joyless and in no mood for celebration. There was profound relief, but even that was qualified by doubt: could it really be true that, for us, the daily struggle to provide blood, plasma and other intravenous fluids, penicillin, sulphonamides, and antimalarials to medical units in Italy, Austria, Yugoslavia, and Greece, had come to an end?

An international team

For two years No 5 Base Transfusion Unit (5BTU) had supplied the Eighth and Fifth Armies; the Americans on the Anzio beachhead and for the invasion of southern France; Tito's partisans by sea and parachute; and also the victims of the tortured liberation of Greece. Around 200 000 service men and women had been blood grouped; blood had been collected from over 75 000 of them and, together with some 95 000 bottles of plasma, 150 000 bottles of glucose/saline, and 165 000 bottles of other solutions and distilled water, had been distributed daily by "the blood plane" or by road up to distances of 450 miles from our main base in Bari to the various fronts.

A small established unit of two officers and 11 men, with one truck, had necessarily grown into a highly irregular one of nearly 200 men and women – British, Canadian, New Zealand, Indian,

173

Polish, and Italian – with at least 40 vehicles acquired in a variety of ways, and with the use of one or two DC3 aircraft. Few of the team had had previous training in any aspect of the equipment or in the science and art of resuscitation; they included members of the Friends Ambulance Unit, VADs, soldiers considered unfit for further fighting duties, and many civilians. Every recruit was welcome; not one of them proved to be a "dud". I learned for all time that everybody can do, and enjoy doing, at least one thing very well. All of them picked up the enthusiasm which many of us had inherited from Lieutenant Colonel G A H Buttle and his forward officer, Keith Lucas, in the middle east. From Tripoli in Libya, through Sicily, Italy, and Austria, to the associated campaigns in Yugoslavia, Greece, and southern France, 5BTU was the base supply depot for up to 19 field transfusion units, each consisting of a medical officer, two or more orderlies, and a driver; an FTU would be strengthened when fulfilling an additional forward distributing role on a particular front.

The group won one OBE, four MBEs, and 14 "mentions", but the record would have been even more impressive if the authorities had not returned my final list, with advice to raise and expand upon my original recommendations – and then totally ignored them all.

One of the lessons Buttle had taught us was that whole blood must be administered in forward surgical units if appropriate surgery under adequate anaesthesia was to be carried out soon after wounding. Plasma was of great value but, contrary to official opinion in the UK, was insufficient for this task on its own. Generally, in the Central Mediterranean Force 10–12% of wounded required transfusion, each man receiving on average, during his whole treatment, 4 "pints" of blood, 5 of plasma, and 6 of glucose/saline. But one Canadian unit, with 40 abdominal cases among its wounded at one time, used 700 bottles of plasma in a single day.

It was astonishingly difficult to put over the idea of "replacement" of just what was estimated to have been lost, whether cellular or fluid. Surgeons often found it difficult to accept the advice of an FTU resuscitation expert. When American surgeons at Anzio were emerging from their tented theatres and examining and re-examining the wounded, Captain Pitt-Payne (OC, 12FTU) hit on the idea of putting up a borrowed blackboard on which he quoted the odds in favour of operation; soon the Yanks were excitedly shouting, "Frank, who's the favourite?" and cheerfully accepting his experienced advice. In all, 5BTU supplied 16 000 bottles of blood to the beachhead.

The UK objection to the use of whole blood was based on fears about its safety. We found the blood grouping noted in pay books or on "dog tags" wildly inaccurate and grouping sera from England almost useless. We had to make our own high titre sera, and were then able to group 200 people an hour, with a subsequent error on rechecking the donated blood of less than 0.3%. An American pathologist at Anzio told a visiting British general that British blood was awful, "giving lots of reactions", but then admitted that he had been there only a few hours and had not seen a single case himself. He readily agreed to make careful notes of the administration of the next 100 bottles of blood and honestly reported, later, that he had noted a reaction in one case only, a transient rise of temperature to 104°F. Four FTU officers who were able to keep careful records reported 6.2% reactions on 3739 bottles of blood, most of them limited to shivering and a rise of temperature below 103°F. No evidence was found of the transmission of hepatitis, and only one case of transmission of malaria.

Wet plasma, however murky in appearance, was remarkably free from reactions. Lack of supplies of wet plasma for landings and parachute drops forced us at one time to reconstitute some 20 000 tins of dried Canadian plasma which we found on a dockside in north Africa. We filtered it all, removing remarkable quantities of fat. On hearing of this the War Office forbade us to do it, and a reply was sent saying that we would stop as soon as other supplies came to hand, but no reactions to the reconstituted plasma were reported.

Trickery, greed, and torture

The first American blood donors downed our beer, and then rather roughly demanded cash in order to "get some dames" – they were led by a doctor, to whom we were indebted for so blatantly revealing the risks of offering payment. After an argument we agreed to certify that they had offered blood, and left it to their pay officers to shell out or not. Very soon after VE Day an agitated general showed me a demand by the US army for repayment of $75 000; I suggested that they should be asked to say what proportion of blood had been given to British wounded, for which

175

we would gladly pay, and not to Americans, Indians, Poles, French etc. Nothing more was heard.

It was exciting, at times demanding and even heartbreaking, to be responsible for penicillin distribution – to those who could be returned to battle. I did not consider that one of Tito's political commissars came within this definition. A Polish hospital called for excessive supplies on the grounds that they had many cases of syphilis (2.4 megaunits per case). On visiting the hospital I found the records of thrice hourly injections complete; I arranged that the adviser in venereology should drop in unexpectedly, but he could only conclude that the Poles had been unlucky in their amorous adventures. Not long after VE Day Polish officers clamoured for war against the Soviet Union; I was then in Trieste and I told them I thought it would be 20 years at least before any Briton would take up arms against the Soviet ally who had suffered such horrendous losses; however, so brutal were the activities of communists in that region at the time that a few weeks later I would have volunteered to lead the Poles. Eventually it came out that, for the most patriotic reasons, the whole of the staff of the Polish hospital had conspired to sell penicillin on the black market in order to equip themselves for the battle against Russia. When that was seen to be impossible there had been a share out according to rank, and two majors admitted to me that they had each bought two villas in Rome.

Whenever the issue of capital punishment arises, I think of a group of American deserters who collected empty penicillin phials, put curry powder or pepper into them, and sold them to frantic Italian parents. I should like to have shot them, but I would never ask someone else to do it for me.

Dropping blood and plasma into Yugoslavia had its rewarding moments but brought revelations of unbearable atrocities. On the good side, the New Zealand surgeon Lindsay Rogers once told me of the miracle of finding a parachute basket full of blood bottles after his forest hospital had been overrun by the Germans, and when he was in despair what to do for the few wounded they had been able to drag away through the woods. On the bad side, there was the crediting, by the political commissars, of all we could supply to the Russians, and the refusal of the British authorities to agree to threaten to cut off all supplies of arms, transport, food, clothing, and medicines by a certain day unless the partisans ceased treating their chief practical allies as enemies – in my view, a healthy and essential step. At the level of abiding sorrow, there were the eye witness accounts of torture, mutilation, and casual death; I was told we could stop this if we declared and dropped leaflets to the effect that after the war every German known to have been in a certain place at a certain time would be executed without trial. I protested that we were fighting for the rule of law, but I often think I was wrong.

Towards the future

It was experiences of this kind which made it difficult to celebrate VE Day. Also I had fallen in love with a partisan woman doctor and was wondering, if I could ever enter Yugoslavia, would I find her alive? (we have now been together for nearly 40 years).

There had been one source of hope for the future: that in the CMF we had worked with people from 12 different nations and had learned to accept them, and to be accepted by them, on personal and not national merit. Elston Grey-Turner, with his proficiency in French and German and his forthright kindness, was one of the not too many British doctors to have a high regard for international friendship. Experience of war did not have to be a total loss in the years afterwards.

During the evening of VE Day a wildly happy bunch of New Zealanders burst in as we were having dinner in rather glum silence; they lined up and performed their *haka* with exuberant enthusiasm. I felt ashamed not to be as blessedly thankful as they were. The sense of shame turned my thoughts at last towards the future and opportunities which had suddenly and unexpectedly become possible.

Elston Grey-Turner*

FERGUSON ANDERSON

I have been given the honour of paying tribute to my friend of many years Dr Elston Grey-Turner. The son of a distinguished surgeon, he was educated at Winchester and Trinity College, Cambridge, and qualified at St Bartholomew's Hospital in 1942. An appointment as house surgeon was followed by his four years' service with the RAMC, initially as regimental medical officer with the 2nd Battalion the Coldstream Guards, in north Africa and Italy, where he was awarded the MC for rescuing the wounded under fire at Monte Cassino. He ended his war career as a lieutenant colonel on Field Marshal Montgomery's staff in Germany, where he met his future wife Lilias. He never lost his affection for the RAMC and continued to serve as an officer in the Territorial Army after the war, gaining the TD and holding an appointment as honorary colonel.

After brief spells in general practice and hospital, and after passing the Civil Service examination with a diplomatic career in mind, he joined the staff of the Ministry of Health and often sat in the officials' box in the House of Commons when Nye Bevan was the minister. His presidency of the Cambridge University Medical Society, his experience in the workings of government, and his remarkable ability as a linguist were to be of great value to him in his future career. In 1948, two months before the inception of the National Health Service, he was encouraged by the then secretary of the British Medical Association Dr Charles (now Lord) Hill, to become an assistant secretary of the association. As overseas secretary Elston Grey-Turner organised a successful action by the doctors of Malta, and later fought for equal pay and opportunity

*From the address given at a service of thanksgiving, St Pancras Church, London, 7 March 1984.

for women doctors in Hong Kong. The special register for professional bodies already carrying out industrial relations work was his idea and this solved the problems associated with the Industrial Relations Bill. Always a great believer in cooperation with the trade unions, he was elected vice chairman of the staff side of the Whitley Council. His gift for languages was of great value in his negotiations with the standing committee of doctors of the European Community, of which he became secretary general.

In 1976 Dr Grey-Turner was appointed secretary of the BMA and was outstandingly successful. He transformed the association by planning regional extensions, thus forging links with individual doctors, and in short created a modern management structure. He also established an economic research unit, and his clear supervision of the BMA's evidence to the Royal Commission on the National Health Service and on the preparation of legislation to reform the General Medical Council was invaluable. In the year of his appointment as secretary he was elected master of the Society of Apothecaries and in this high office revealed his great gifts as host and raconteur. In 1980 his qualities of loyalty, honesty, friendship, and kindness to all resulted in his election as a vice-president of the association; his awards of a CBE, an honorary MD, the Queen's Jubilee Medal, appointments as an honorary physician to the Queen and as an officer of the order of St John were among the many honours given so justly to him. He was also chairman of the medical board of the St John Ambulance, a fellow of the Royal Society of Medicine and a member of the Honourable Artillery Company. Perhaps his proudest moment was when he was invited to deliver the Grey-Turner memorial lecture, established in memory of his father, to the International Congress of Surgery in 1979 in San Francisco.

Throughout his memorable career Elston was supported on every occasion by his loving and lovable wife, Lilias. In the acknowledgements of the *History of the British Medical Association. Vol II: 1932–1981*, written jointly by Elston Grey-Turner and F M Sutherland, appears the following: "We are profoundly grateful to our wives for their infinite patience and forbearance when they discovered that our retirement from the staff of the BMA, at any rate to the present, has been an illusion."

Elston Grey-Turner was not cast in the common mould – a man of patrician appearance with finely drawn features, he was constantly aware of his social conscience. Other people's problems were always in his mind and too often regarded as his fault. His war experiences had left a deep and lasting impression and he was sometimes haunted by the thought of the loss of the flower of a generation. He had shown to all his bravery in battle, his calmness in true crisis and his ability to make lasting friends. He had an impish sense of humour, with sudden bursts of laughter, and his membership of the Ombrellino club, consisting of reunions of veterans of the Italian campaign, revealed the lighter side of his nature. He delighted in the formal dinner, revelled in the correct order of precedence, in a well organised parade, and in the continuity of tradition. He was very proud of his father and of his army connections and loved his beautiful home. He knew everybody worth knowing – showing this, for example, in his relations with the palace. When he was asked to organise a meeting of the World Medical Association in London, receptions, accommodation, and entertainments were laid on at the drop of a hat.

During his time of service to the BMA he devoted his whole life to his work. No one was ever more friendly or better loved by the staff, and this extended from the elite few to those with the most menial tasks. All were known by name. Elston was the perfect English gentleman, cultured, with a sound classical education, always charming, never too busy to talk to anyone, and as straight as a die. As secretary his door was ever open – any unhappiness among his staff became his problem. Service has been defined as giving a little bit of oneself to others and Elston gave almost too much. He was generous in the extreme, completely without rancour and always fair; advice given by Elston was good advice.

He described the most moving ceremony of his life as the dedication by the Archbishop of Canterbury of the World War II memorial at BMA House in 1954, and it was noted that he was deeply moved whenever he visited a Commonwealth War Graves Commission Cemetery on his foreign tours. His sense of history was revealed by his great pleasure at the RAMC dinner in 1976, when the late Lord Mountbatten sat at his right hand reminiscing about his boyhood days with the last Tsar and Tsarina of Russia.

Elston's life was guided by two maxims. The first is a saying from Mark Twain: "Always do right; this will gratify some people and astonish the rest." The second the advice of a Dr William Cowan: "Be pleasant to people; you may often find this difficult but nevertheless be pleasant. You cannot know what secret mental anguish they may be suffering."

To me Elston was first a soldier of honour and then a doctor. His staff called him, with great affection, "The Colonel" and Bunyan's words ring true:

> Who would true valour see,
> Let him come hither;
> One here will constant be,
> Come wind, come weather.
> There's no discouragement
> Shall make him once relent
> His first avow'd intent
> To be a pilgrim.

My feelings of affection for Elston will always remain. I loved him for his zest for life, his complete integrity, his pride in morale and in his country, and his delight in tradition. He sought and fought for a better world for all and inspired others with his devotion to duty and by the warmth of his personality. Let me conclude with these lines which recall for me his delight in conversation and his lovable nature.

> I wept as I remembered how often you and I
> Had tired the sun with talking and sent him down the sky.

f-6.00